Focused Clinical Assessment in 10 Minutes for MRCGP

Featuring data-gathering, clinical management and communication skills

DR ISRAR KHAN

MBChB, MRCGP, DCH, DRCOG, DFSRH

Foreword by

DR ROGER NEIGHBOUR OBE

Radcliffe Publishing

London • New York

Radcliffe Publishing Ltd
33–41 Dallington Street
London
EC1V 0BB
United Kingdom

www.radcliffepublishing.com

British Library Cataloguing in Publication Data

A catalogue record for this book is available from the British Library.

ISBN-13: 978 184619 974 5

The paper used for the text pages of this book is FSC® certified. FSC (The Forest Stewardship Council®) is an international network to promote responsible management of the world's forests.

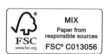

Typeset by Beautiful Words, Auckland, New Zealand
Printed and bound by TJ International Ltd, Padstow, Cornwall, UK

Contents

Foreword

In real life, once your general practitioner (GP) training is completed and you've passed the Membership of the Royal College of General Practitioners (MRCGP) assessment, a typical consultation lasts anything between 5 and 15 minutes. In real life, some consultations go well and others not so well, and that's okay. In real life (let's be honest), you can sometimes bluff your way out of a tricky situation, or play for time. And in real life, the patients are real patients, not simulated, and they don't come in followed by a silent observer clutching a clipboard and looking inscrutable yet vaguely threatening.

But if you're a GP registrar over whose head (and bank account) the Clinical Skills Assessment (CSA) looms ominously, you may find yourself slipping into a parallel universe in which what passes for real life is very different. In CSA-dominated practice, every consultation lasts 10 minutes, exactly 600 seconds. In those 600 seconds, you must infallibly identify the patient's stated and hidden agenda, not forgetting to explore their ideas, concerns and expectations. You must skilfully perform a selective but focused clinical examination. You must formulate a management plan that accords with every known guideline, while allowing the patient to share in its creation. All this you must not only do, but must also make sure that the person with the clipboard sees that you do, 13 times in straight succession.

It seems that in the CSA candidate's alternative nightmare version of reality, you mustn't put a foot wrong. Or so you may fear. And if this is what you think is expected of you, you are probably suffering from a new but epidemic syndrome – CSA-related consultation dysfunction (CCD).

People like me, to whom assessors are no longer a threat, are fond of advising – and it is still good advice – that the best way to prepare for the CSA and prevent CCD is to spend at least 6 months beforehand developing and practising your consulting skills until sorting out whatever your patients bring you becomes almost natural. Then, on the day, go into the CSA and consult like you always do. But the sufferer of CCD develops selective amnesia for this advice. In the grip of CCD, a young GP experiences a craving for structure, for a system, for scripts and stock phrases. Under the stress of assessment, consultations can become stilted and formulaic. The victim of CCD tends to lapse into the hospital-acquired doctor-centred *'if you ask enough closed questions, you won't miss anything'* mode, which is almost guaranteed not to elicit the unique features of an individual patient's story.

The essential skills needed for a good GP consultation are not hard to describe. My friend David Haslam, who succeeded me as Royal College of General Practitioners (RCGP) president, summed them up succinctly: *'Shut up. Listen. Know your medicine. And care.'* In other words, pay close attention to your patients. Be curious about them. Help them talk freely. And listen to what they tell you. Talk to every patient as one intelligent, sensitive and valuable human being to another.

Ah, but how? That's easy to say, but not so easy to do, let alone to learn, and especially to learn for an exam.

True. That's where this book will be so useful. It really does help to bridge the gap between meaning to consult in a patient-centred way and actually coming out with the right words at the right time motivated by the right reasons. CSA candidates in particular will find plenty of sound advice about how to manage those all-important 600 seconds – active listening, data gathering, focused examination, decision sharing and the rest – but in a way that keeps the bigger picture constantly in mind; namely, to have the patient leave your consulting room having been genuinely helped by spending 10 minutes with you.

I take my hat off to Dr Israr Khan. It is encouraging and somehow affirming to find a young colleague who understands so well the key subtleties of the consultation and who can put them across so helpfully to CSA candidates who also need a steer through its minutiae. Dr Khan's experience of the exam is still sufficiently fresh to give his advice valuable credibility.

So buy – read – study – this book. All I would say is, don't leave it too late. Dr Khan can help you translate good intentions into real-life words and actions. But only if you give him time. Start learning from him months before your exam. If you wait until the week before, not even he can rescue you.

In real post-CSA life, a consultation style such as Khan's will help you acquire your best insurance against frustration, burnout or blunting of your sensitivities. So thank you and congratulations, Israr. And good luck to you, his readers. Enjoy your careers in this most fascinating of medical specialties.

Dr Roger Neighbour
OBE, MA, DSc, FRCGP, FRCP
Bedmond
April 2012

Preface

I have written this book with one principal aim: to provide you with a unique structure for the focused clinical assessment and management of everyday problems encountered in general practice, in 10 minutes. I see this book as an extension to my working life and something of excellence that I am particularly proud of. Writing this book provided me with a fabulous opportunity to help general practice specialty trainees thrive. Personally, I am thrilled that I have been successful in completing the book, and I hope it guides and benefits all GP trainees.

Dr Israr Khan

MBChB, MRCGP, DCH, DRCOG, DFSRH

Walsall

April 2012

About the author

The text of this remarkable book has been written in a comprehensive yet straightforward style through the hard work and dedication of a recently qualified practising GP, Dr Israr Khan. Dr Khan graduated from the University of Birmingham Medical School in summer 2006, with subject honours in pathological studies and therapeutics. After completing the 2-year foundation training programme in Sandwell in 2008, he joined the 3-year Vocational Training Scheme of Blackcountry North, West Midlands, successfully completing the scheme in 2011.

He is now a role-model GP in Walsall with a real love for working in general practice, enjoying the diversity, the unique relationships and the challenge of dealing with the unknown. He enjoys his specialist interests in minor surgery and child health surveillance, and has a deep passion for the delivery of medical education, to both undergraduates and postgraduates.

Acknowledgements

This book is the result of the exceptional hard work and indefatigable efforts of a handful of enthusiastic people from many spheres of life. I recognise the outstanding contributions of medical and non-medical contributors involved in shaping this book and am further grateful for their support and influence.

I would like to thank Dr Roger Neighbour, former president of the RCGP, an MRCGP examiner for over 20 years, and author of the classic text books *The Inner Consultation* and *The Inner Apprentice*, for writing the Foreword. I have found the work of Dr Neighbour immensely illuminating, and there is no doubt, either, that he has been extremely influential.

I am particularly grateful to my sister, Farzana Idrees, a dedicated biomedical scientist in Walsall, for her helpful comments and feedback.

I am delighted to acknowledge, with sincere thanks, my closest friend, Dr Shahid Merali, a talented, energetic and popular GP in Birmingham, for his continuing inspiration and encouragement. Dr Merali's instrumental involvement from the book's earliest beginnings has been integral to its success. Drafts were regularly sent to Dr Merali for his in-depth reviews, constructive critique, useful advice and editing, and I would like to express my gratitude to him for his invaluable input.

My special thanks also extend to Mrs Janet Hughes, a retired English teacher and friend, who has made an enormous contribution in helping with the editorial process.

Finally, on a personal note, I would like to offer my sincere appreciation and thanks to my dearest wife, Sofia Tabassum, for her everlasting support and patience during the lengthy but remarkably rewarding journey of this book.

This book is dedicated to my dearest parents for their endless love, continued support and ongoing encouragement. Thank you, Mum and Dad.

List of abbreviations

ADL	activities of daily living
BP	blood pressure
CSA	Clinical Skills Assessment
DM	diabetes mellitus
DIY	do-it-yourself
DVLA	Driving and Vehicle Licensing Agency
DH	drug history
FH	family history
GMC	General Medical Council
GPST	General Practice Specialty Training
GP	general practitioner
HPC	history of presenting complaint
ICE	ideas, concerns and expectations
MRCGP	Membership of the Royal College of General Practitioners
NICE	National Institute for Health and Clinical Excellence
NRT	nicotine replacement therapy
OCP	oral contraceptive pill
OTC	over-the-counter
PMH	past medical history
PIL	patient information leaflet
PC	presenting complaint
PSA	prostate-specific antigen
PSH	psychosocial history
RCGP	Royal College of General Practitioners
SIGN	Scottish Intercollegiate Guidelines Network
TB	tuberculosis

Introduction

Focused Clinical Assessment in 10 Minutes for MRCGP aims to equip the reader with the knowledge, understanding, skills and attitude required for effectively structuring a focused GP consultation in 10 minutes and developing a successful consultation style for the CSA. It has been written specially for General Practice Specialty Training (GPST) registrars at any stage of their training, especially those at the beginning of their first GP placement, and for CSA candidates. But all practitioners, however experienced, are likely to benefit from this book.

This book provides a step-by-step guide describing the essential components of the consultation, followed by a systematic, ordered approach for structuring a 10-minute consultation, helping you to handle successfully any problem encountered in general practice. It places a huge emphasis on a frank and fluent approach for taking a targeted history and performing a selective clinical examination of the patient (i.e. gathering information as part of the focused clinical assessment), and presents a systematic framework for formulating and sharing diagnoses and management plans with patients.

This book also introduces you to the key communication skills and techniques that are available to enhance data gathering, gain an understanding of the patient's illness experience and share information with patients effectively.

Various communication skills techniques to employ during the professional interview – in particular, appropriate questioning styles and counselling techniques – are presented. Examples of useful questions to ask patients to gather relevant data, when to ask these questions, how to ask these questions sensitively, how to explain examinations correctly, how to communicate investigations/results/diagnoses and how to negotiate sensible management options with patients, in the right way, are all provided.

Finally, dealing with difficult patients, conflict between patients and doctors, ethical dilemmas and medico-legal issues can be extremely challenging for the doctor. A constructive and practical approach to tackling some of the most difficult and complex consultations encountered in general practice is also presented to familiarise you with the consultation strategies required to manage such cases. The challenging consultations include such situations as managing patients demanding antibiotics for self-limiting viral illnesses, assessing risk of self-harm, counselling patients for specific investigations, through to breaking bad news and conflicts of interest regarding driving and epilepsy.

Chapter 1

About the MRCGP

This chapter contains details of the formal summative assessments that comprise the MRCGP assessment programme. Since September 2007, there has been a single compulsory training and assessment system for UK-trained doctors wishing to obtain a Certificate of Completion of Training in General Practice. Satisfactory completion of the scheme is an essential requirement for entry to the register of GPs maintained by the General Medical Council (GMC) and for the MRCGP.

The MRCGP is an integrated training and assessment strategy that reflects the complete mix of knowledge and skills required for competence in general practice.

The MRCGP assessment has three essential components:

1. A workplace-based assessment

This is a placement-based competency assessment using an e-portfolio to collect evidence throughout the GPST programme. This assembled evidence needs to be submitted towards the end of your final specialist training year.

2. Applied Knowledge Test

This is the summative assessment of the knowledge base that underpins independent and safe UK general practice. It is a multi-choice-question exam paper taken during the second year of the specialist training programme (ST2). It comprises 200 questions in various formats: true/false, best from five and extended matching (best from many). Approximately 80% of the questions will focus mainly on various aspects of clinical medicine and therapeutics, 10% on critical appraisal

3

and evidence-based practice (research and statistics) and 10% on administrative, ethical and legal issues.

3. CSA

This is the clinical consulting skills examination and can only be undertaken during the third and final year of the GP specialist training scheme (ST3). It serves as a summative test for end-point assessment in order to determine whether the candidate has reached the required standard expected of a newly qualified GP.

Each of these components is independent and assesses different aspects of knowledge, understanding, skills and attitude as applied to general practice, but together they encompass the entire curriculum for UK specialty training for general practice.

Chapter 2

Overview of the CSA

The CSA is an essential component of the MRCGP, and is '*an assessment of a doctor's ability to integrate and apply clinical, professional, communication and practical skills appropriate for General Practice*.'[1]

The MRCGP CSA is a challenging examination of a young doctor's performance in a patient consultation. The CSA aims to test a wide range of clinical and non-clinical skills in an objective fashion. The main aim of the examination is to assess whether a candidate has reached the standard in clinical skills expected of a newly appointed, competent GP who is in the final stages of completing GPST.

To prepare for the CSA, it is useful to understand what is being assessed by the exam. The CSA examination is designed to assess a doctor's ability to gather relevant information and apply learned understanding of disease processes and person-centred care appropriately in a standardised context, to make evidence-based decisions and to communicate effectively with patients and colleagues. Although up-to-date working knowledge of general practice and of general medicine is necessary to pass this assessment, it is not primarily a test of theoretical knowledge and understanding. It is a test and measure of your ability to integrate and apply clinical and communication skills to the specific scenarios, to produce a consultation that is meaningful to both patient and doctor, and which moves the patient forward towards a justifiable management of their presenting problem. In order to do well, you need to demonstrate different aspects of good consulting.

The CSA assesses your ability to:

◆ Take a focused, yet holistic history

◆ Perform a targeted clinical examination

◆ Assimilate information from the 'patient notes' and integrate that into the consultation

◆ Evaluate and interpret the clinical findings of the history and examination, and identify key issues in the data gathered

◆ Establish a working diagnosis/differential diagnoses

◆ Formulate a safe, shared and acceptable management plan

◆ Communicate this information effectively to patients

This makes up the complete knowledge set, skills and attitude expected of CSA candidates, and this book will cover all of these areas in detail.

Candidates are expected to demonstrate proficiency in the following areas:

◆ History-taking, carrying out physical examinations and using diagnostic instruments (i.e. performing a focused clinical assessment of the patient)

◆ Assessing symptoms and signs accurately and integrating these findings

◆ Clinical judgement (diagnosis and management) reflecting information gathered during data gathering

◆ Knowledge and understanding of common and serious medical conditions in UK general practice

◆ Communication – targeted information gathering and information sharing and giving

◆ Professional behaviour

◆ Ethical practice

The CSA exam

During the CSA examination session, you will see 13 patients, all of which are assessed and contribute to the overall final mark. Each consultation will be limited to 10 minutes, followed by a 2-minute resting gap where you have the opportunity to read carefully the case material in preparation for the following consultation. The beginning and end of consultations will be signalled by a buzzing sound.

At the start of the assessment, the buzzer will sound and the first patient will knock and enter the candidate's consulting room. At the end of 10 minutes, the buzzer will sound again to mark the end of the consultation, and the patient will leave the room, along with the examiner. This process will be repeated until all 13 cases in the surgery have been seen. There is a designated 15-minute break approximately halfway through the assessment circuit.

Domains of performance

The three equally weighted domains of performance (also known as consulting competencies) assessed in the CSA are:
1. Data-gathering, technical and assessment skills
2. Clinical management skills
3. Interpersonal skills

You should appreciate that the CSA is not just a test of your communication skills but is a comprehensive exam testing your clinical knowledge, understanding, practical skills and attitude as applied to general practice. Excellent doctor–patient communication and interpersonal skills alone are not enough. It is not correct to assume that if you are a good communicator you will pass the exam, as two-thirds of the marks reflect two other clinical areas (data gathering and clinical management). Competency in all three clinical domains is essential, as the overall mark given to a case will depend on the candidate's ability to combine the two areas of clinical consulting with communication and interpersonal skills.

The next three chapters provide further details of the three domains of performance on which you will be marked during the CSA. In turn, they deal specifically with these domains in a GP surgery consultation and can easily be adapted to fit the telephone triage or domiciliary settings. They have been devised to inform candidates about the core data-gathering (history-taking and examination), clinical management (which includes diagnosis and appropriate treatment/referral) and interpersonal (including communication) skills required for competence in these domains of performance.

Chapter 3

Data-gathering, technical and assessment skills

The first of the three domains of performance assessed in the CSA is **data-gathering, technical and assessment skills**, also known as data-gathering, examination and clinical assessment skills:

Gathering and using data for clinical judgement, choice of examination, investigations and their interpretation. Demonstrating proficiency in performing physical examinations and using diagnostic and therapeutic instruments.

Areas of the curriculum assessed by this domain are **problem-solving skills** and **clinical practical skills**.

Problem-solving skills:

Gathering and using data for clinical judgement, choice of examination, investigations and their interpretation. Demonstration of a structured and flexible approach to decision-making.

Clinical practical skills:

Demonstrating proficiency in performing physical examinations and using diagnostic and therapeutic instruments.[1]

Introduction to data-gathering skills (focused clinical assessment)

The data-gathering skills section of the CSA is about gathering relevant and focused information from history-taking, clinical examination and results of investigations (provided in the case notes) for clinical judgement, identifying significant abnormal findings in the data gathered, appropriately evaluating and interpreting the clinical findings and, finally, recognising their implications and significance.

In simple terms, data gathering tests your ability to take a targeted history, perform a selective clinical examination (to elicit physical signs) and gather information as part of the focused clinical assessment of the patient. Then, later on in the consultation, the data collected should be used to establish a working diagnosis or consider a limited list of possible differential diagnoses, formulate a safe and acceptable management plan and communicate this information effectively to the patient.

Data gathering, particularly history-taking, also tests your ability to use appropriate communication and interpersonal skills to gather information more effectively. Therefore, there is a degree of overlap between these two domains of performance assessed in the CSA examination.

A focused clinical assessment is the cornerstone for managing symptoms and clinical conditions in general practice. Being able to make good clinical decisions depends on gathering and making the best use of valuable information from a focused clinical assessment. GPs need to be able to perform a focused clinical assessment using organisational and clinical skills at a high level, often under time constraints, to manage their patients safely and appropriately. The two essential components of the focused clinical assessment are taking an accurate history and carrying out a selective physical examination, in a patient-centred way. Assessing patients clinically through history-taking and physical examination provides the basis for safe and effective clinical practice. This chapter will clearly guide you through a focused clinical assessment of a patient in a systematic and efficient manner.

It is divided into the following three sections:

3.1. History-taking

3.2. Performing a physical examination

3.3. Interpreting results of investigations provided

3.1. History-taking

The CSA assesses your ability to take a focused history, assess symptoms and signs accurately and identify the key issues in the presentation.

You will be expected to take a history accurately and sensitively from the patient or carer that routinely includes biological, psychological and social factors.

By the end of history-taking, you need to have a full understanding of the problem or dilemma presented and its implications for the patient.

The following sub-sections will systematically take you through history-taking in some detail. They concentrate on gathering important and relevant information from a focused history and clinical examination and assessment of the patient.

3.1.1. Background

The consultation (the professional interview) is absolutely basic to the job of the GP. By this stage in your training, you may be feeling comfortable in the consultation setting. An important part of consulting is the development of basic clinical skills, which include taking a patient history. The history in the GP consultation is a very powerful tool to deal with the majority of problems encountered in everyday practice. Exact figures vary, but there is general agreement that the majority of diagnoses may be reached on the basis of history-taking alone; that is to say, merely by talking to the patient.

By this stage in your training, you should be taking competent histories naturally and easily and have developed an appropriately professional style. In the CSA, you will have to take a concise, relevant, targeted and systematic yet comprehensive and holistic history of the presenting symptom/problem that includes all the relevant information required for making a working diagnosis/list of possible differential diagnoses, identifying appropriate investigations to confirm the diagnosis and formulating a safe management plan.

3.1.2. Introduction

At the beginning of the assessment, the buzzer will sound and the first patient will knock on the candidate's door and enter the consulting room, along with the examiner. Stand up, gently smile, make good eye contact and shake the patient's hand. Greet and welcome them politely into the consultation, using their name (the opening greeting) and clearly introduce yourself, using your professional title and surname. Starting with a good, solid introduction often helps to put patients at ease.

3.1.3. Open consultation: presenting complaint (PC) – open questions

The consultation should start with an initial open-ended question to attempt to discover the main reason(s) for the patient's attendance (i.e. to identify patient's agenda). An 'open question' is one which cannot be simply responded to with a one-word or one-phrase answer; it is formulated to engage the person answering, and to allow them to express themselves according to the question, to gain as much information as possible. Open questions are particularly helpful to find out the reason(s) for a person's visit and to spot a hidden agenda or a potential ethical dilemma. They are most useful at the beginning of the consultation because they increase the chances of identifying relevant problems early in the consultation. For example, questions such as, *'How can I help you today?'* or *'What can I do for you today?'* can elicit the reason(s) for the patient's contact, their PC or their concern(s) more easily. Use a phrase that you feel comfortable with and that sounds natural and caring.

Eliciting the patient's main problem(s) is a key task in communicating with patients that good doctors should be able to perform. Doctors frequently interrupt patients soon after they begin their opening statement, with patients failing to disclose their complaints and/or concerns fully. Listen patiently to the patient's initial narrative, and be able to obtain an accurate description of their presenting problem. Expect them to do most of the talking early on, and don't interrupt the patient until they have disclosed their PC or voiced their concerns.

Once you have identified the reason(s) for the consultation, follow up with a second open and probing question to address the patient's agenda, fully exploring the nature of the presenting problem. For example, *'Can you tell me a little bit more about that, please?'* Give the patient time to gather their thoughts and bring up other aspects of their complaint.

If you are ever stuck in the CSA, other useful open questions that can be used to facilitate the doctor–patient dialogue and elicit more information include: *'Tell me how it all started?'*, *'How long has it been going on for?'* and *'If you go back to the day it started, can you tell me exactly what happened?'*

Therefore, the three simple but essential open questions that can be helpful in the CSA are:

1. *'How can I help you today?'*
2. *'Can you tell me a little bit more about that, please?'*
3. *'Can you tell me how it all started?'*

3.1.4. The 'golden minute'

In order for you to identify the patient's hidden agenda and recognise significant verbal and non-verbal patient clues (signals or messages), we have something called the 'golden minute'. This is a very critical time at the beginning of the consultation when a great deal of valuable information can be elicited. During the golden minute, allow the patient to do most of the talking, pay close attention to what they tell you and be alert to unconventional as well as conventional medical clues you receive from the patient. Allow the patient to say what they want freely, encourage them to tell their individual story in their own words and give them a chance to disclose their concerns, perceptions and feelings about their predicament.

Avoid unnecessary interruptions that interfere with dialogue or rapport (unless you absolutely have to). The advantage of saying nothing is that it allows you to listen to the patient's version of the problem, in their own words. This is at the heart of the contemporary fashion for narrative-based medicine: *'Listen to the patient: they are telling you the diagnosis'*. Listen actively to what the patient actually says, pick up on the patient's agenda (which may be hidden), emotions and worries (if they are evident) and respond to them with genuine interest and sincerity. Responding to emotional clues with various communication strategies enhances further disclosure. Listen attentively to the patient's story to ensure that clues in the consultation that require your full attention are not missed. Often by listening, key issues will be disclosed that would never be found by closed questions. For example, the symptomatic presentations of sore throat, cough, abdominal pain, etc. will have different underlying stories that will not be so obvious with a history taken by closed questioning. (Don't underestimate the level of challenge presented by the apparently trivial complaint or underestimate the complexity of apparently simple consultations.)

Aside from listening to what your patient actually says, you need to be constantly aware of non-verbal signals. Observe the patient and look at their non-verbal communication. You can become alert to such facial indicators as frowns, raised eyebrows and blushes. Picking up on and responding appropriately to the patient's clues, both verbal and non-verbal, is a key component of patient-centred interviewing. Using relevant information gained from acting on patient clues is likely to increase patient satisfaction and adherence to treatment, and lessen patient vulnerability to anxiety and depression.

Finally, throughout history-taking, be encouraging, nod your head while listening, lean forward, make good eye contact and say *'mmm'*, *'yes'*, *'sure'* or some other emollient phrase at appropriate times to facilitate the dialogue progression.

3.1.5. History of presenting complaint (HPC) – closed questions

When assessing a patient clinically, the main bulk of the consultation should be spent on collecting information in a focused yet patient-centred way. You will need to demonstrate proficiency and competence in obtaining an adequate history from the patient, recognising the importance of focusing on the patient's problem(s).

A focused yet comprehensive assessment of the PC is clearly central for recognising and managing symptoms in general practice. The history should initially focus on the relevant issues around the patient's current PC and underlying condition (address the patient's agenda) with a series of closed-ended questions. Closed questions are the most efficient method of obtaining further details about a patient's problem and help clinch details of the clinical history. For example, *'Where exactly is the pain?'* or *'When did the pain start?'*

Use selected closed questions mainly to assess the nature and duration/time course of the PC, to clarify the patient's answers and to explore pertinent symptoms from the relevant system(s) to differentiate various possible diagnostic lines. Further points to be determined should appear to be guided by the probabilities of disease. You need to know the important and relevant questions to ask for different symptoms competently and confidently and be able to follow up various possible diagnostic lines. Questions should be phrased simply and clearly, and double or misleading questions should be avoided. If you ask good questions, you will get good answers, and if you ask poor questions, you will only get poor answers.

What the patient says or does may change your subsequent line of thinking and questioning approach. Therefore, keep an open mind, don't make immediate assumptions about the problem and don't have any preconceived ideas about what it may be. Be led by what the patient wants to talk about and address the patient's agenda. Don't be occupied in thinking about what you are going to say next and miss what the patient is saying now or what s/he is doing. Don't just have the next question ready in your head; if you do, your history-taking will appear disjointed, with your line of questioning erratic and not following a clearly reasoned way of thinking. The consultation will appear disorganised and unnatural, as some elements will be thrown in apparently at random. Rather, be appropriately selective in the particular questions you ask, embedding your enquiry in previous responses, so that a fluent and logical progression is clear. The consultation should have a clear sense of progress, and matters should be advanced as a result of the consultation.

Finally, avoid using formulaic phrases in your questions that are not normal for everyday consulting. Relying on stock phrases that do not suit your individual style of consulting can sometimes be perceived as an interrogation, as the open questions rapidly turn to closed biomedical history-taking. Adopting a non-interrogative and non-threatening approach to history-taking allows patients to come forward about their problem(s) more comfortably and openly.

3.1.6. Red flags/Alarm symptoms

The other main issue to consider when assessing patients clinically is the identification of important and relevant red flags (or alarm symptoms), which are worrying features specific to each condition. Systematically searching for important symptoms and being aware of their implications can help identify diagnoses that you should try not to miss and increases the chance of diagnosing more serious disease, such as cancer, earlier.

Red-flag questions can help to rule in and rule out potentially serious organic pathology and ensure the consultation is safe. Red flags are very unlikely to be known beforehand or offered spontaneously by the patient and have to be elicited. If an important red flag is missed and therefore an unlikely but serious disease is not ruled out, it may be seen as unsafe and dangerous. This does not mean that you have to go into every conceivable detail or chase rare diagnoses. It is about taking a patient history in the degree of detail that is compatible with safety but which takes account of the epidemiological realities of general practice.

3.1.7. Patient health beliefs, understanding and preferences: ideas, concerns and expectations (ICE)

All patients have different health beliefs: ideas (thoughts/perceptions/feelings), concerns (worries) and expectations, influenced by personal experience, media information or family/cultural beliefs. Doctors rarely ask their patients to volunteer their ideas about their problems and, in fact, doctors often evade their patient's perceptions and inhibit their expression. Yet, if discordance between doctor's and patient's ideas and beliefs about the illness remains unrecognised, poor understanding, adherence, satisfaction and outcome are likely to ensue.

Enquiring about the patient's ICE shows responsiveness to their health beliefs, health understanding and health preferences and effectively demonstrates patient-centred consulting. ICE lie at the heart of patient-centred interviewing and should be gathered in the first half of the consultation. Sometimes the health beliefs of patients will be obvious in a consultation, sometimes not. Patients don't always come forward with their own ideas, thoughts, perceptions, feelings and concerns about their predicament, and sometimes have to be prompted or asked about them directly. On occasion, they may volunteer their health beliefs without any prompting. Sometimes, the way they look or what they say gives you clues to an underlying worry, and you should develop the necessary skills to recognise these behaviours.

For most cases in the CSA, it is important to ensure that you enquire about all the patient's health beliefs properly and sufficiently at some point in the consultation, using ICE questions in a realistic way, where appropriate for that case, so you can use the information gathered to guide the rest of the consultation. Details of the patient's ICE do not need to be investigated exhaustively, but the patient's perspectives of a problem should be sought and you should have a clear idea of any ICE.

When to ask about the patient's ICE will vary depending upon the PC. Examples of ICE questions include:

+ I: *'What do you think might be causing it?'*

+ C: *'Is there anything about what's going on that's particularly worrying you?'*

+ E: *'What do you hope I will be able to help you with today?'*

When eliciting the ICE of patients, avoid using formulaic phrases in your questions that are not normal for everyday consulting; for example, *'What are your worries?'* Avoid following a scripted approach that feels 'clunky' or insincere to the patient or to the examiner. Be yourself and make the ICE questions you use sound like your own natural speech, not like questions you have heard from others. Also, you are more likely to find out about the patient's ICE if you tailor your questions and their timing to each individual, rather than asking the questions out of context.

Don't forget to address and deal with the patient's ICE later in your explanations. Asking questions about a patient's main concerns, for example, but then not utilising the information or integrating it into the consultation does not demonstrate person-centred care.

3.1.8. The rest of the medical history

Gather the rest of the medical history in sufficient detail, covering all the relevant aspects of the case. Work through the routine history in a logical manner enquiring about relevant past medical history (PMH), past surgical history and previous hospital admissions; drug history (DH), including over-the-counter (OTC) medications, herbal remedies and drug allergies; and family history (FH), if appropriate to the circumstances presented.

History-taking is not expected to be all inclusive, and so this does not have to be done in every consultation to ensure that no information has been left out. With this in mind, do not take too long to cover what is not thought to be essential, as it can lead to poor time management, and only enquire about relevant history that you might find helpful as part of your focused clinical assessment of the patient. Remember that it is about obtaining sufficient information about symptoms and details of the medical history, tailored to the circumstances, which in turn defines the clinical problem(s).

3.1.9. Psychosocial history (PSH)

The patient's social and cultural background has an effect on personal definitions of, beliefs about and attitudes towards health and disease, and also has an effect on their response to illness. An understanding of the impact of social factors upon health and sickness and the role of psychological factors as determinants of disease and health is required.

Demonstrating an awareness of the impact of health problems (acute or chronic illness, hospitalisation or the death of a patient/relative) on the patient's life, their perception of themselves, their relationships and their family is central to practising effective patient-centred medicine.

Patients come to the doctor with problems that have clinical, social, psychological and emotional dimensions. Doctors have a responsibility to consider all aspects of a patient's well-being, including biological, psychological and social factors. You will be expected to recognise the social and psychological factors contributing to each consultation (what non-clinical issues have prompted the patient to consult). You will need to think beyond the biomedical model of disease and recognise the effects that social factors may have on the patient's illness and vice versa, and appreciate the importance of psychological factors for patients and their families.

Where appropriate, as part of your extended data gathering, it is necessary to elicit the relevant social background and psychological aspects of the presentation to place the patient's problem in context. It is essential to explore the physical, psychological and social impact of the patient's problem on their everyday life rather than just their health to establish a complete picture of their PC. What impact does the illness have upon the patient's personal and social lifestyle, including the ability to function at work, home and leisure activities? What effects does the health problem have on the patient's image? What are the effects of the illness on the members of the patient's family? Exploring these areas is very important for maintaining a therapeutic relationship and a therapeutic environment in community settings. They show the patient that you are interested in his or her psychosocial well-being and that of the family. Additionally, you will find building up a personal understanding with the patient very rewarding in everyday practice.

3.2. Performing a physical examination

The CSA assesses your ability to perform a targeted physical examination (to elicit physical signs), demonstrate appropriate clinical examination skills and interpret clinical signs.

You will be expected to examine patients accurately and sensitively in appropriate settings to gather relevant data.

3.2.1. Background

An integral part of focused clinical assessment and data gathering is to carry out a physical examination, where appropriate, especially if it would be useful in establishing the diagnosis. The main aim of the physical examination is to rule in your working diagnosis and to rule out other potentially serious underlying conditions that have entered your differential diagnoses. Also, by performing an appropriate examination, you show that you take the person seriously and that you care, which can help with establishing rapport. Having said this, clinical examinations are not the main basis of the assessment, and are infrequently tested in the CSA. More commonly, the assessor or the patient will give you the physical findings of an examination after you have sought permission to perform it instead of agreeing to the examination.

3.2.2. Approach to the clinical examination of the patient

After a history has been taken from the patient, a few cases will require the patient to be examined and some clinical examination skills to be demonstrated. Don't leap quickly to less productive physical examinations without appreciating the importance of a good, adequate history. Taking a well-organised history will give you a solid basis for guiding your physical examination (and making clinical judgements). Use the information that you gather to plan your physical examination and think of which signs you would look for so that you can adopt a focused and selective examination.

Before carrying out any physical examination, the patient's permission must be sought and a simple explanation given. If the patient feels that a proposed examination would be personally intrusive, they will decline the examination.

Always offer the patient a chaperone; male doctors will require a chaperone when examining female patients in many circumstances, female doctors in certain cases. In the case of intimate examinations, you should make absolutely sure you have gained informed consent and offered a chaperone. These are examinations that you are unlikely to be asked to demonstrate on a role player, but a mannequin or model may be used in the consultation to demonstrate a clinical examination technique.

At all times during the physical examination, show sensitivity for the patient's feelings and be alert to non-verbal clues. Undertake the examination in a way that does not distress the patient.

You will not normally find abnormal physical signs when conducting clinical examinations, but you should examine the patient in such a way that you would elicit them if they were present.

On completing the physical examination, don't just leave the patient, but assist them getting off the examination couch, getting dressed, etc. if you feel help is needed. Don't forget to wash your hands after each patient is examined. Usually, an alcohol hand gel is provided on the desk in each consultation room. Performing this task is also part of being a successful candidate.

3.2.3. Diagnostic equipment

You will be expected to be knowledgeable, proficient and competent in the appropriate use of standard clinical instruments and in examination techniques, including use of a stethoscope, ophthalmoscope, auroscope/otoscope, thermometer, patella hammer, tape measure and peak flow meter. This includes having an understanding of the appropriate use of these medical devices in common situations. Again, your technique needs to be smooth and fluent, as if you use them regularly and you use them well.

3.3. Interpreting results of investigations provided

The CSA assesses your ability to analyse and interpret the results of methods used in the investigation of common and serious medical conditions in primary care, and to recognise their implications and significance.

You should be able to analyse and interpret test results accurately. These include such results as urinalysis, urine microscopy, culture and sensitivities, swabs, bloods, electrocardiographs, X-rays (e.g. chest radiographs), scans (e.g. ultrasound), spirometry and skin scrapings.

The results of investigations may be provided in the 'patient's notes', and you may find some of this information useful to integrate into the consultation. It is therefore absolutely essential to read all the background information relating to each case before the patient enters your consulting room.

Further on, the data collected during the clinical assessment phase of the consultation should then be used in the clinical management stage of the consultation to establish a working diagnosis/construct a limited list of possible differential diagnoses, formulate a safe and appropriate management plan and communicate this information effectively to the patient.

Chapter 4

Clinical management skills

The second of the three domains of performance assessed in the CSA is **clinical management skills**:

> *Recognising and managing common medical conditions in primary care.*
> *Demonstrating a structured and flexible approach to decision-making.*
> *Demonstrating the ability to deal with multiple complaints and co-morbidity.*
> *Demonstrating the ability to promote a positive approach to health.*

Areas of the curriculum assessed by this domain are **primary care management** and a **comprehensive approach**.

Primary care management:

> *Recognising and managing common medical conditions in primary care.*

Comprehensive approach:

> *Demonstrating proficiency in the management of co-morbidity and risk.*[1]

Introduction to clinical management skills

The clinical management skills section of the CSA is primarily about the diagnosis and management (including appropriate investigations, therapies and referral) of common and serious medical conditions in primary care.

A sound understanding of the range of common and serious medical problems presented to doctors in general practice and the range of preventative, investigative and therapeutic options available is necessary for this particular domain to be done well.

Candidates should carefully synthesise, evaluate and interpret evidence objectively from the patient's medical history, physical examination/mental assessment of the patient and results of any investigations provided, to make the most likely diagnosis or generate a limited list of possible diagnoses. Then, on the basis of the clinical findings and working diagnosis, formulation of plans for management should be made using further investigation, community-based resources or referral to other services as appropriate, valuing the opinion of the patient and their significant others, and matching the investigation and treatment plan to the patient's and/or their carer's wishes.

Making a diagnosis from clinical findings, formulating a sensible shared management plan, which takes into account best practice, and giving information to patients about diagnosis and management are the most difficult parts of the CSA. This chapter will effectively guide you through the appropriate and sensitive clinical management of a patient.

It is divided into the following two sections:

4.1. Diagnosis

4.2. Management

4.1. Diagnosis

The CSA assesses your ability to establish an appropriate working diagnosis or construct a limited list of possible differential diagnoses reflecting the information gathered (during data gathering) using your clinical diagnostic skills. It is also designed to test your ability to share and discuss a diagnosis with the patient simply, clearly and sensitively.

You should be able to use relevant information obtained during data gathering to draw appropriate conclusions, establish a specific diagnosis or range of diagnoses and communicate this information accurately and effectively to the patient.

4.1.1. Clinical knowledge

Although the CSA is not a test of medical knowledge, it does require a good clinical knowledge base and its application across the broad range of UK general practice. An excellent breadth of knowledge and clinical skills and a level of sophistication with which the knowledge base is contextualised and applied appropriately to clinical situations is necessary to be able to confidently establish and communicate the working diagnosis.

4.1.2. Making a diagnosis/differential diagnoses

The main purpose of performing a focused clinical assessment is to be able to define the usefulness of the information collected to formulate appropriate differential diagnoses and rule out serious underlying illness. Making a diagnosis includes assessing patients clinically through taking a careful history, carrying out an appropriate clinical examination, assessing symptoms and signs accurately, considering a list of possible differential diagnoses and identifying appropriate investigations to confirm the diagnosis.

A common reason for running out of time in CSA cases is candidates spending far too long taking a history and then having to rush the second half of the consultation, the clinical management phase. A frequent sign of poor consulting skills is a candidate who puts off making a diagnosis or clinical decisions, thus running out of time in the consultation to go through the management options properly. You should think carefully about all the information that is presented in the case and organise your thoughts. The exam requires you to evaluate and interpret the clinical findings of the history and examination, and investigations provided, if any, to identify the key problems and formulate a working diagnosis (or a limited list of possible differential diagnoses). Common and serious primary care clinical conditions should be considered in the differential diagnoses, remembering that common things occur commonly and are more likely than uncommon ones in real life, as well as in the CSA.

4.1.3. Explaining the diagnosis

Conducting an effective patient-centred consultation also involves sharing information with patients. With this in mind, a clear explanation of the probable clinical diagnosis should be conveyed to the patient in an adequate and confident way, involving them in the discussions where appropriate. Focus your explanations on the diagnosis, the causation and the prognosis of the condition. You will need to be knowledgeable and confident in the facts about the illness in order to be able to give advice appropriately.

There must be appropriate tailoring of the amount and type of information given, so that you achieve a shared understanding of the problems with the patient. A short explanation about the findings and problem may be enough, but it must be relevant, understandable and tuned to the patient in an appropriate language, without the use of jargon or inappropriate technical descriptions that the patient might not understand.

When imparting clinical information, the patient's level of knowledge and understanding of medical and health matters should be established and your explanation should be appropriately adjusted to these. Share your thoughts and ideas in a manner that patients and relatives understand, and assess their comprehension using appropriate non-verbal communication.

Explanations are often most effective when you affirm a patient's health beliefs. You should tailor your explanations of the diagnosis to demonstrate an understanding of the patient's health beliefs, essentially by a reference back to the patient-held ICE. This ensures you remain patient-centred throughout your 10-minute consultation.

4.1.4. Checking patient understanding before moving on

After the explanation, you should make a discreet digression to check how well the information has been understood. It must be an active seeking process to confirm that the explanation has been understood and accepted by the patient. If the patient does not appear to understand, you should pick this up and reformulate your explanation.

4.2. Management

The CSA assesses your ability to devise a safe, shared and acceptable management plan to deal with common and serious primary care problems. It is also designed to test your ability to negotiate and share a management plan with the patient simply, clearly and sensitively.

You will be expected to formulate a plan of action, appropriate to the findings, in collaboration with the patient, and communicate this to the patient accurately and effectively.

You will need to demonstrate a sound understanding of the range of prevention, investigation and treatment options available in primary care.

4.2.1. Clinical knowledge

One of the feedback statements commonly given by examiners to CSA candidates is: *'Does not develop a management plan (including prescribing and referral) reflecting knowledge of current best practice.'*[1]

An understanding of the clinical management of the problem(s) presented is also a test of your working knowledge base underpinning common and serious medical conditions seen in UK general practice. Sufficient knowledge, understanding and skills are required to be able to integrate and apply theoretical knowledge appropriately to facilitate the management of common physical, psychological and social problems seen in primary care. Your knowledge of medical management in relation to general practice should be of a very high level, and you will be expected to put forward realistic and detailed treatment plans. You need to have the knowledge, understanding and skills to manage problems competently and safely in primary care in a way that reflects good current best practice. You will therefore need to feel confident in the facts about the management of the illness in order to be able to give advice appropriately. You need to be familiar with up-to-date national clinical guidelines and protocols in general practice, such as those published by the National Institute for Health and Clinical Excellence (NICE) and the Scottish Intercollegiate Guidelines Network (SIGN) to be able to think of a range of such management options. Clinical management should be evidence based and linked to recognised algorithms or modes of practice, as suggested by NICE, SIGN or other national guidelines. Also, your understanding of decisions for referral to other services or a specialist should be in line with current guidelines and best practice.

4.2.2. Negotiating and sharing management

Person-centred consulting partly involves sharing information with patients and agreeing on a sensible management plan. Having said this, *'Finding common ground to develop a shared management plan where relevant, in partnership with the patient'*[1] (a feedback statement), is one of the areas that most candidates find difficult in the CSA. It is the single most common reason for candidates failing a case.

Candidates should devise a sensible and feasible plan of action, appropriate to the findings, in collaboration with the patient. The patient should be involved in significant management decisions, agree on the plan of action and be encouraged to accept appropriate responsibility. This respects that the patient is the expert in their experience of their illness.

Genuinely negotiate management of a problem with the patient. Empower and support patients to make appropriate choices for themselves, and respect their decisions. It is not uncommon that candidates can sustain a patient-centred consultation style for the data-gathering part of the consultation but then easily switch to a doctor-centred mode in 'telling' the patient what they should do or take. Take special care not to instruct the patient; rather, you should offer sensible and feasible management options (if there are options) for the situation in hand, and provide relevant information on these appropriately. This allows the patient to engage in shared decision-making, respects the individual's autonomy, maintains patient-centredness and displays empowering behaviour.

The best shared management plans take account of the patient-held ICE gathered in the first half of the consultation, incorporating these into the explanation given to the patient about their diagnosis as well as using them to guide the patient through the appropriate management options for the problem(s) presented.

4.2.3. Formulating management options

You will be expected to demonstrate your clinical problem-solving skills competently, recommending a range of reasonable management options to the problem(s) presented (when options are available) that are likely to be tailored to and acceptable to the patient. Importantly, the underlying management plan should relate directly to the working diagnosis, must mirror good current medical practice and take account of the patient's views to aid the development of shared understanding.

The management options offered should include the things that the patient can do themselves to manage their symptoms, the things that you can offer that are likely to be agreeable to the patient and, finally, the things that the patient may need to refrain from if their problem/diagnosis is likely to render them a source of danger to themselves or others, such as work, driving, heights, activities, etc.

4.2.3.a. Things the patient can do themselves: lifestyle modification

The sorts of things that the patient can do themselves to manage their symptoms are mainly to do with non-pharmacological aspects of management, so relevant advice about changes in lifestyle, such as diet (general and specific), smoking cessation, limiting alcohol consumption, exercise and weight loss, should be given. It is important to determine the patient's perspective before discussing lifestyle changes.

4.2.3.b. Things you can offer the patient: biopsychosocial model

When planning the sorts of things that you can offer to manage the patient's problems, the biopsychosocial model is a useful guide to demonstrate your ability to think of realistic and effective alternatives. You should be familiar with both pharmacological and non-pharmacological aspects of management.

The biological treatment choices you may recommend include conservative measures, for example, watchful waiting/wait and see: using time as a diagnostic and therapeutic technique is unique to GPs, lifestyle advice, relaxation exercises, physiotherapy, acupuncture, etc.; therapeutic measures (OTC drugs and prescription-only medicines); surgical interventions such as joint injections and minor/major surgery; or appropriate referral (routine, urgent or emergency/same day) to other services (community or hospital).

Psychological management methods you may suggest include relevant advice and support from various professionals, talking therapy, counselling and cognitive behavioural therapy (CBT) – combination of face-to-face, telephone and guided computerised CBT, etc.

Social interventions you may suggest include referral to a smoking cessation advisor/clinic, referral to the alcohol intervention team, referral to social services, appropriate advice on time off work (e.g. provide a sick note/medical certificate) or relevant advice on informing the Driving and Vehicle Licensing Agency (DVLA), if appropriate to the circumstances.

Solutions to problems should be discussed openly, so that the patient fully understands the implications. The patient should be guided through the different treatment options, making them aware of the relative risks (adverse effects and complications) and benefits of the different approaches. Your role as a doctor is to give the patient the opportunity to be involved in significant management decisions by providing basic counselling and advice on the facts, benefits and potential harms of each sensible option, so they can make an informed decision. Patients who take part in decision-making are more likely to adhere to treatment plans.

It is worth stating that it is not enough that you know how to manage a problem; you must show the examiner that you know how to do this. You cannot obtain marks for unspoken thoughts. You need to make the management plan explicit to the patient, so that the examiner is satisfied with what you are planning to do and why. Your agreed plan of management for the individual patient must be adequate enough to satisfy the examiner that you are a safe practitioner and have managed the problem(s) appropriately and sensitively.

4.2.3.c. Things the patient may need to refrain from

Bear in mind that you may need to give the patient relevant advice or instructions about things they should refrain from if their problems/diagnosis may put them or others at risk of danger or harm; for example, driving, cycling, swimming and climbing ladders/scaffoldings/trees, etc.

4.2.4. Further investigation

If appropriate, candidates should choose and instigate reasonable further investigations – for example, midstream urine, blood tests, imaging – justify the appropriateness of the investigation(s) requested, be able to request the investigation(s) and be able to explain to the patient exactly what will be done. Further tests should be ordered to help establish or confirm a diagnosis and to rule in or rule out a disease, often in response to red flags, and when a diagnosis does not fit any pattern of disease. Candidates should ensure that they request diagnostic testing judiciously, only requesting investigations if they are likely to affect their management. It is bad practice to instigate a battery of tests as this will make you appear indiscriminate.

4.2.5. Health promotion

Prevention and health education are issues that should be thought about in every consultation. It is considered good practice for GPs to take opportunities as they arise to give patients relevant advice on ways in which they can improve their overall health; for instance, by stopping smoking, increasing exercise or reducing alcohol intake. Health-promotion activities demonstrate a rounded view of healthcare and an awareness of the importance of maintaining the patient's health.

There needs to be sensitive and appropriate handling of health promotion. Gathering data for health promotion is important and relevant, but firing off a list of health-promotion questions out of context is unlikely to be welcomed by the patient and is less likely to be effective. Also, giving very brief lifestyle advice, for example, if the consultation finishes early, in order to 'tick the box', is deemed inappropriate.

It is important that you promote good health at opportune times in the consultation so that it complements the patient's agenda. The key to doing this successfully is to identify the patient's health beliefs and work with them towards a plan for maintaining good health. Another way is to appropriately link the relevant health promotion to what the patient came in for. For example, if a patient who is a smoker presents with worsening asthma, you could sensitively link smoking to their asthma exacerbation to encourage smoking cessation. This also demonstrates effective use of the consultation.

4.2.6. Summarising

There are significant problems with patients' recall and understanding of the information that doctors impart. The evidence suggests that periodic revision of the main points of an explanation is positively related to patient understanding and recall. For example, one way that a doctor can increase compliance is to repeat the important parts of the instructions. Summarising at appropriate times can also help demonstrate a fluent approach.

4.2.7. Safety-netting

It is important for all patients to know when they should come back if their illness has not improved. 'Safety-netting' is a term that describes the specific explanations that should be given to each patient about what to expect, including a timescale if appropriate, and about what to do if symptoms get worse or develop in some way that is unexpected. Effective safety-netting ensures a contingency plan has been made for the worst-case clinical scenario and that the consultation is safe. A clear description of where and how to get help, at any time of day or night (if this seems appropriate for the issues being presented), should be included.

4.2.8. Follow-up

A consultation should not be seen as an isolated incident but rather part of the continuum of the course of an illness. Making arrangements for follow-up demonstrates your commitment to the continuity of care of patients and your concern for their welfare and safety. It shows that you are prepared to take responsibility for managing the ongoing presentation of the condition until the problem has been resolved in some way.

You should have a very positive attitude to follow-up and be prepared to make timely arrangements for the patient, when appropriate. Necessary arrangements for follow-up that reflect the natural history of the problem should be planned appropriately to the level of risk. Timescales for follow-up as to when you will see the patient again should be clearly specified.

4.2.9. Further information

You can enhance the consultation in a patient-centred way by providing additional useful information containing important diagnostic, prognostic and safety-netting advice, as well as evidence with regard to pharmacological and non-pharmacological treatments that you may have recommended.

Offer the patient relevant information through patient information leaflets (PILs) or direct them to a well-known website, such as those of the British Asthma Society, the British Heart Foundation and the British Diabetic Association (Diabetes UK), or to a more general website, like Patient UK, where they can search up-to-date medical information. If you offer to give a PIL, you will only gain marks if you have explained the contents of the written material.

Knowing about the various agencies, both statutory and voluntary, that can provide support to patients and their families in coping with their health and/or social problems is also useful – for example, social services, Age UK, Citizens Advice bureaux, Alcoholics Anonymous, Quitline and Cancer Research UK.

4.2.10. Take responsibility for any gaps in understanding shown by the patient

In the final stages of the consultation, you can also take responsibility for any gaps in understanding shown by the patient in order to spare their anxiety over appearing slow or stupid. The wording of this is very important: saying *'Is there anything I have said that I have not been clear about?'* is better than, *'Is there anything you didn't understand?'* Although having essentially the same meaning, the first does not demean the patient in any way, where the second might be taken as an insult to their intelligence.

4.2.11. Deal with any extra issues

Ask about any extra complaints only when you have finished dealing with the patient's PC. Don't go hunting for extra problems or issues at the beginning of the consultation. Also, don't deal with extra problems before you have adequately dealt with what the patient came in for.

Most patients in the CSA will only have one problem. If the patient has two problems, they are both likely to be simple complaints. Occasionally, there may be a case where the patient presents with multiple health problems, both acute and chronic. In these types of clinical scenarios, it is important to construct a problem list and prioritise. Remember that you do not have to achieve everything in a single 10-minute consultation. You have the option to use time and to review the patient at a later stage as appropriate.

4.2.12. Close consultation

Summarising the main points is a useful technique to use when achieving closure of the consultation. There should be a shared understanding before the patient leaves your room, and this can be confirmed by asking the patient to summarise what they have understood. Alternatively, you can summarise the salient points that you want the patient to remember.

The consultation should then be terminated (usually by the doctor) using a closing farewell.

4.2.13. Housekeeping

Housekeeping was described by Roger Neighbour's five consultation tasks/ checkpoints in his book *The Inner Consultation*.[2] It refers to clearing the mind of the psychological remains of one consultation to ensure it has no detrimental effect on the next.

After each consultation, try to refresh your mind and move on to the next case with your full concentration and with equanimity. Going over a bad case in your mind may affect your performance in the next. In the CSA, this might mean having a minute to yourself to recover from an emotionally draining consultation.

Chapter 5

Communication and interpersonal skills

The third of the three domains of performance assessed in the CSA is **interpersonal skills**:

Demonstrating the use of recognised communication techniques to gain understanding of the patient's illness experience and develop a shared approach to managing problems. Practising ethically with respect for equality and diversity issues, in line with the accepted codes of professional conduct.

Areas of the curriculum assessed by this domain are **person-centred care** and **attitudinal aspects**.

Person-centred care:

Communicating with patient and using recognised consultation techniques to promote a shared approach to managing problems.

Attitudinal aspects:

Practising ethically with respect for equality, diversity and the patient's view point, with accepted professional codes of conduct.[1]

Introduction to communication and interpersonal skills

The interpersonal skills section of the CSA is primarily to do with effective doctor–patient communication.

The CSA assesses your ability to communicate and consult with patients of different ages and from different social backgrounds and with different intellectual capacities in a highly professionally acceptable manner.

You will be expected to communicate appropriately with patients throughout consultations, whether it be through simple history-taking, counselling on some aspect the patient is unclear about, sharing information or giving advice.

Background

The art of communication for doctors is perhaps the most important part of practising medicine. Whether communicating with patients, colleagues or relatives, it is what sets the great doctors apart from the good. It is what patients remember most: how you talked to them, how you interacted with them, how you treated them, whether you identified their main problems and their perceptions about their predicament, whether you gave them a chance to air their concerns and whether you took their worries on board.

Good communication skills are essential for maintaining a high standard of patient care. The success of many doctor–patient relationships depends on our ability to communicate effectively. When doctors use communication skills effectively, this has several benefits for their patients. Doctors with good communication skills identify their patients' problems more accurately; their patients will disclose more concerns, perceptions and feelings about their predicament; their patients are more satisfied with their care and can better understand their problems, investigations and treatment options; their patients are more likely to adhere to treatment and to follow advice on behaviour change; and, finally, their patients will feel less distressed and their vulnerability to anxiety and depression will be lessened.

Effective communication and interpersonal skills are hugely important within the medical profession. The general public and our patients have high expectations of our medical prowess and our communication skills. We will never meet everyone's expectations, but the skill and effort that we put into our clinical communication does make an indelible impression on our patients and their families.

Anyone who wants to be regarded as a good doctor needs to possess effective communication skills. Poor communication lies at the heart of patient dissatisfaction and can lead to a patient's belief that they have received poor care. Current evidence shows that a lax attitude towards communication can have serious professional and legal implications for doctors. Poor communication skills have long been established as a major risk factor that can lead to complaints from patients against doctors and have been shown to be a predictor of burnout.

The GMC emphasises in *Tomorrow's Doctors* that doctors should be able to '*communicate clearly, sensitively and effectively with patients and their relatives, and colleagues from a variety of health and social care professions*'. The GMC regards the ability to communicate effectively as being a core clinical skill. It is therefore essential to teach and test this in the same way as other clinical subjects.

Some people make the assumption that communication is 'inherent' and therefore underestimate the complexity of clinical communication and its centrality to effective practice. It was a commonly held belief that communication skills could not be taught – that they were natural talents and inborn attributes of the good doctor – and a young doctor was either endowed with them or not. It has traditionally been difficult for many doctors to accept the idea that something as supposedly intuitive as communication could or should be influenced by teaching or training. Everyone expects doctors to be good communicators, but the truth is that good communication is often quite difficult, and further training is essential to enhance our communication abilities. Communicative and interpersonal skills are technical skills that can be learned, and the doctor who lacks them can be said to be lacking in technique, in the same way as the doctor who lacks clinical knowledge. Effective communication skills teaching and training therefore plays an essential role when preparing for the CSA to ensure that you acquire the skills necessary to communicate well with patients.

This chapter will effectively guide you through the key clinical communication and interpersonal skills and techniques required to consult well with patients in everyday general practice. It explores the skills essential for effective communication with patients and discusses how to acquire these skills. It contributes specifically to the development of appropriate skills in interviewing and communication required for success in the CSA.

It is divided into the following two sections:

5.1. Non-verbal communication skills

5.2. Verbal communication skills

    5.2.1. Gathering information

    5.2.2. Information sharing and giving

Some of the topics covered here should also complement the notes in the data-gathering chapter, Chapter 3, which has relevance to communication skills.

Communication skills

Throughout your consultations, you will be required to demonstrate an understanding of the components of effective verbal and non-verbal communication skills. Entire books have been written on communication and consultation skills, but in-depth knowledge of the various models of consultation is not required to pass the CSA. The following two sections highlight the basic, generic skills needed for effective non-verbal and verbal communication with patients. They provide some straightforward practical pointers to incorporate flexibly into your communication with patients that may well help you to communicate more effectively.

5.1. Non-verbal communication skills

This section aims to improve your background knowledge and understanding of the basic concepts required for effective non-verbal communication with patients.

Dress code

When you attend the assessment centre, be tidy in your appearance and dress appropriately. In general, casual clothes, such as denim jeans, sloppy jumpers, crop tops and other fashion items are not acceptable.

Professionalism

At all times, appear professional in your approach and interact appropriately with patients. Establish and maintain a friendly but professional relationship with patients throughout consultations. If you don't have good professional relationships with your patients, you will achieve much less. You need to develop a manner and approach that earns you the respect and confidence of patients.

Attitude

Be polite, respectful, understanding and helpful; you'll be far more convincing if you are reasonable and courteous. Have the right attitude, show interest in the patient, and treat them with kindness, compassion, consideration and in a non-judgemental manner, without prejudice. Show patience and sensitivity in your communications with patients, and recognise that your general conduct and manner count towards being a good GP.

Skills

High-standard communication and interpersonal skills should run throughout consultations. A good interviewer is one who stays calm, relaxed and interested throughout the consultation, and makes the patient feel relaxed and at ease. You should be able to connect instantly with the patient, achieve a good working relationship quickly and pick up the patient's agenda early on. You should engage and develop a general rapport (and trust) with the patient early in the consultation and maintain this rapport throughout. Rapport is about building a connection on a human-to-human level rather than a doctor-to-patient basis. This is not possible in every case but is helpful to the doctor–patient relationship.

Show a genuine interest, even a curiosity, about the patient that is open, non-judgemental and caring in nature. Have warmth in your voice, manner and approach. Have a positive attitude when dealing with problems such that the patient would feel they would wish to see this doctor again.

Be aware of personal space and maintain an appropriate doctor–patient distance. The gap should not be too close, whereby the patient is intimidated, but not too far, whereby it looks as if you're not interested. Also, be on the same level as your patient (your chair should not be much higher).

Be curious about the patient. Show that you care and that you want to find out what's really going on. Through your body language, signal to the patient that you are interested in them as a person. For example, put your pen down, face the patient, meet the patient's gaze, smile and nod your head at appropriate times. Use facial expressions appropriately, for instance, frowning, and hand gestures when explaining something, keep an open body posture, lean forward when appropriate and give them your undivided attention. Establish eye contact at the beginning of the consultation and maintain it at reasonable intervals to show interest. Maintaining eye contact may be uncomfortable, but it is an important way of establishing rapport. Avoid crossing your arms, as this shows you're 'closed', uncomfortable, nervous and insecure, and in turn the patient also closes down and doesn't want to open up. Instead, rest your arms on the table or on your lap.

The interviewee should do most of the talking, and you should actively listen to what the patient says and how they say it. Often by listening, key issues will be disclosed that would never be found by closed questions. *'The most important thing in communication is to hear what isn't being said'* (Peter Drucker). In other words, listen with your ears, eyes and brain, and listen to what is said and what is not said.

Aside from listening to what your patient actually says, you need to be constantly aware of non-verbal clues and respond to them with genuine interest and sincerity. For example, if the patient appears anxious, then you could respond appropriately by saying, '*You seem very anxious*'. Picking up (and responding appropriately) to patient clues is a key component of patient-centred clinical method.

5.2. Verbal communication skills

Various communication skills and techniques are available to use to find out about the reason for a patient's attendance, gather data effectively, gain an understanding of the patient's illness experience and take a shared approach to managing problems. This section aims to improve your background knowledge and understanding of the basic skills required for effective verbal communication with patients. It specifically expands on the key verbal communication and consultation skills necessary for gathering information and information sharing and giving.

5.2.1. Gathering information

As we have seen, data gathering is a very powerful tool to deal with the majority of problems encountered by doctors. This section goes through the essential communication skills and techniques necessary to gather information from patients, with particular attention paid to the questioning skills required to elicit this information.

The following communication skills (and strategies) and questioning styles to enhance data gathering will be addressed in turn:

5.2.1.a. Questioning styles: open, closed, leading and multiple question types

5.2.1.b. Useful prompts

5.2.1.c. Explaining to the patient what you are doing

5.2.1.d. Enquiring about sensitive/embarrassing information

5.2.1.e. Normalising statements

5.2.1.f. Clarification

5.2.1.g. Demonstrating empathy using reflection

5.2.1.h. Reassuring the patient

5.2.1.i. Silence

5.2.1.j. Summarising

Questioning styles (open, closed, leading and multiple questions) are basic but essential communication skills necessary to gather information more effectively from different patients, whereas normalising statements, clarification, reflection, appropriate use of silence and summarising are more advanced interview techniques. Together, they are some of the essential communication skills and techniques that contribute to good consulting behaviour and style in the CSA.

5.2.1.a. Questioning styles: open, closed, leading and multiple question types

A successful interview consists not only of well-prepared questions but also good interviewing techniques. During data gathering and clinical assessment, your task is to use appropriate questioning skills to elicit relevant information from patients. The information you collect should include identifying the main reason(s) for the patient's attendance (finding out why the patient has come to the doctor today), relevant issues around the PC, the patient's ICE (exploring what the patient is worried about and what they expect from the doctor's appointment) and appropriate psychological and social information to place the problem in context. The quality and relevance of the information you gather should be used to inform further questions and move the consultation forward in a meaningful way.

Various questioning styles, such as open-ended and closed-ended questions are available to employ during the professional interview to gather information most effectively. Your consultations must show evidence of the use of appropriate questioning techniques to gather information from patients.

Open questions

Open questions are far more effective than other question formats for gathering information. An open question is one which cannot be simply responded to with a one-word or one-phrase answer; it is formulated to engage the person answering, and to allow them to express themselves according to the question, to gain as much information as possible.

This strategy can be particularly helpful for discovering the main reason(s) for the patient's attendance and to spot a hidden agenda or a potential ethical dilemma. Open questions also help to identify psychological or social issues, which will often be useful for putting the presenting problem in context.

Some examples of useful open questions:

'What can I do for you (today)?'
'Tell me, what seems to be the problem?'
'Can you tell me a little bit more about that, please?'
'Tell me how it all started?'
'How did it all begin?'
'What do you mean by a "funny turn"/"dizzy spell"/"dizziness"?'
'Have you had any thoughts as to what might be causing it?'

'Is there anything about what's going on that's particularly worrying you?'

'Have you had any thoughts as to what I might be able to do for you today?'

'Why do you want this X-ray really badly?'

'What do you think the antibiotics will do?'

'How is the pain affecting your life?'

'How are things at school/college/university/work/home?'

Closed questions

Open questions are useful for identifying issues important and relevant to the patient, which you can then illuminate further with the use of more closed (direct and specific) questions. A closed question can be responded to with a one-word or one-phrase answer, although the person answering can expand further if they want to; it is formulated to clarify a specific detail, usually after having asked an open question on the subject.

Closed questions are the most efficient method of obtaining further details about a problem presented to help clinch details of the clinical history. They do, however, have the potential to make the consultation less patient-centred or inappropriately paternalistic (doctor centred), and also can result in patients withholding information, but if used appropriately they demonstrate appropriate doctor centredness.

Some examples of closed questions:

'Where exactly is the pain?'

'When did the pain start?'

'Have you had anything like this in the past/before?'

'How often does it occur?'

'How long does it last for?'

'Does the pain spread anywhere or does it stay in the . . .?'

'Have you taken anything for the pain?'

'How bad is the pain on a scale of 0 to 10, 10 being the worst pain you have ever had and 0 being no pain at all?'

Between the opening greeting and closing farewell, there needs to be an appropriate use of open and closed questions. Avoid too many closed questions, particularly at the beginning of the consultation. As a general rule, open questions are most appropriate at the start of a consultation, followed up by closed questions later. Try to adopt a non-patronising approach to closed questioning that appears conversational rather than interrogative in tone.

Only ask one question at a time, and never interrupt the patient with a question (unless you absolutely have to), as it interferes with the dialogue or rapport. The same information should not be asked for repeatedly (repetitive questioning), as it shows you have not listened to the earlier responses. Questions should be phrased simply and clearly, and double, multiple or misleading questions should be avoided.

Leading questions

A leading question is weighted with a bias to suggest a particular answer from the responder. Although they can be useful in particular settings, they are often used inappropriately.

It is best to avoid using leading questions altogether.

Some examples of leading questions:

'You haven't had any chest pain, have you?'

'You haven't passed any blood in your urine, have you?'

Multiple questions

Multiple questions are a series of related questions formulated within one overall question. They can be confusing to respond to accurately, as it is difficult to structure an answer to multiple questions.

Some examples of multiple questions:

'Tell me how and when this began and what's changed since?'

'Is the chest pain accompanied by any shortness of breath, nausea or sweating?'

By and large, if you ask good questions, you will get good answers, and if you ask poor questions, you will only get poor answers. However, like other surface skills, it is not enough to just do the actions. There is little point in asking a good question if you are unable to respond appropriately to, or use and contextualise, the answer given. You need to listen to the patient carefully in order both to inform the next line of enquiry and move the interview on in a meaningful way. Don't be occupied in thinking about what you are going to say next, as you can miss what the patient is saying now or what they are doing, and this can change the whole consultation.

5.2.1.b. Useful prompts

There are several verbal and non-verbal prompts that can be used appropriately to encourage the patient to continue talking, such as head nodding, leaning forward, good eye contact, repeating the last few words the patient says and also straightforward requests.

Repeating the last phrase from the patient's last sentence can encourage the patient to continue their story:

'You said you have tried all sorts of things for the pain. What sorts of things have you tried?'

'You mentioned it is affecting your body in all sorts of different ways. In what different ways is it affecting your body?'

You can also use straightforward requests like:

'Tell me a little bit more about that, please.'

'Can you say more about . . .?'

'It would help me if I knew more about that.'

'Go on.'

'Take your time.'

'Yes, that's right.'

'Mmm.'

'Uh huh.'

'Okay.'

'Sure.' ('Sure' can be taken as a yes when you don't actually mean that, so be careful when using 'sure.')

Prompts can be helpful to demonstrate evidence of active listening to the patient (and to the examiner) and they also acknowledge what the patient is telling you.

5.2.1.c. Explaining to the patient what you are doing

Explaining to the patient what you are doing and why is good for patient care and also demonstrates to the examiners that you have a clear, well-thought out, logical and systematic approach to data gathering. When you intend to use closed questioning to gather focused information, it is sometimes helpful to warn the patient that you will be asking a set of brief and direct questions, which can help them focus. This can be done by using the suggested phrases:

'Is it okay if I ask you a few specific questions about your X?'

'I would like to ask you a few specific questions about your X, if that's okay?'

'Would it be okay if I asked you some specific questions about your X?'

'Would it be okay if I asked you some specific questions now?'

'May I ask you a few specific questions about your X, if that's okay?'

'I'm going to ask you some specific questions about your X, if that's okay with you?'

'In order to rule out/make sure this isn't a serious medical problem, I'd like to ask you a few specific questions, if that's okay?'

5.2.1.d. Enquiring about sensitive/embarrassing information

Likewise, sensitive information should be asked for in a different manner to routine medical symptoms. Signposting to the patient that one is entering a potentially difficult territory is useful:

'Is it okay if I ask you something a bit personal/private/sensitive now?'

'I would like to ask you a few personal/private/sensitive questions, if that's okay?'

'I'm going to ask something a bit personal/private/sensitive now. Is that okay?'

'As it's relevant and may be important, I'd like to ask some sensitive questions, if that's okay?'

If a patient is embarrassed to talk about their symptom, deal with them sensitively:

'The first thing to say is that we see this quite a lot. It's very common. Lots of people of your age have this problem. I appreciate you're feeling embarrassed, but I might need to ask you some personal questions so that we can get to the bottom of

this. Whatever we talk about will be confidential and won't leave this room. There is no need to feel embarrassed.'

5.2.1.e. Normalising statements

Ask all difficult questions with a normalising preface so that the patient doesn't feel it's just them but it's part of everyday routine practice:

'I would like to ask you a routine question that we ask everybody.'

'Sometimes, people feeling like this . . .'

'In this practice, we always like to do the following tests . . .'

Normalising statements also limit patient worry and anxiety.

Here are some examples:

'I would like to ask you a routine question that we ask everybody. Do you ever seem to hear noises or voices when there is no-one about and nothing else to explain them?'

'Sometimes, people feeling like this hear noises or voices when there is no-one about and nothing else to explain them. Has this ever happened to you?'

'Sometimes, when people are feeling low, they have thoughts that perhaps life is not worth living anymore, if it were to continue as it is at the moment. Have you ever had these thoughts/have you ever felt like that?'

'Sometimes, people, when they are stressed, turn to other things to help them cope. Have you noticed this?'

5.2.1.f. Clarification

You should seek clarification of any jargon used by the patient as appropriate, using clarifying questions.

'What did you mean by . . . "funny turn"/"dizzy spell"/"dizziness"/"migraine"/ "depression"/"anxious"/"paranoid" . . .?'

'Is it okay if I go back and clarify . . .?'

5.2.1.g. Demonstrating empathy using reflection

Doctors should develop appropriate relationship-building skills, with particular attention paid to acquiring the ability to communicate empathetically with their patients, to develop an understanding of the patient as a person with individual concerns and wishes. Empathy should be used when responding to certain patient clues – these clues can be verbal or non-verbal. Empathy demonstrates a caring manner, shows the patient that you understand them and that you have some sense of how the patient is feeling.

The actual process of acknowledging and addressing emotions is not impenetrable or esoteric. The central techniques are straightforward, and involve using a process called 'reflection'. Reflection is a really powerful tool used to demonstrate empathy. Reflection is where you suggest an emotion as to what the patient is feeling. In other words, you respond to a significant patient clue by putting into words what you see (i.e. verbalise what you see – just say what you see). So you are not actually saying what the patient is feeling, but suggesting what they are feeling; that is, adding a light question to it. Acknowledging what the patient is feeling comforts the patient. It demonstrates that you care about them, that you are paying attention and that you are listening, and also enables you to connect with the patient.

Essentially, there are two components to the reflective technique (reflection): suggestion and emotion, creating an empathic statement/response. For example, in the reflective statement *'It must be difficult for you'*, *'It must be'* is the suggestion and *'difficult'* is the emotion you have recognised and acknowledged. Several examples of reflective statements (empathic responses) are illustrated following:

'It must be difficult for you.'
'It must have been difficult for you.'

'You seem very anxious/worried/upset/low/angry.'
'You seem to be very upset by that.'
'You seem to be feeling anxious/worried/upset/low/fed up/angry.'
'You seem to be finding it very difficult to describe how you feel.' (This is a very useful reflective statement for an uncommunicative (mute) patient.)

'You look really anxious/down/low/fed up/upset.'

'It looks like you're finding this difficult.'
'It looks like you're feeling really fed up/anxious/low.'
'It looks like you're feeling upset.'

'It sounds like you've had a terrible time.'
'It sounds like you've been through a lot.'

'It's as if you were feeling upset.'
'It's as if you were feeling really fed up/anxious/low.'
'It's as if you're finding this difficult.' (This is a very useful reflective statement for an uncommunicative or embarrassed patient.)

'It's as though you found that hard.'

'I can see this is very difficult for you.' (This is a very useful reflective statement for a tearful patient.)
'I can see this is very distressing for you.'
'I can see that you are upset.'
'I can see that you are upset hearing this news.'
'I can see that you have got quite a lot on your mind.'
'I can see that you are struggling, Mr X.'
'I can see that this has come as an awful shock/surprise to you.'
'I can see this has clearly upset you.'
'I can see that you clearly look really down.'
'I can see that this has caused you a lot of upset.'
'I can see that this seems to have made you very upset/sad/angry.'
'I can see that it upsets you to talk about . . .'
'I can see that hearing the result/news of the scan is clearly a major shock to you.'

'I can only imagine it is upsetting you.'

'I can appreciate that you are feeling upset/sad/anxious.'
'I can appreciate that you are feeling a lot of pain and discomfort.'

'I wonder if you were feeling very upset/guilty.'

Avoid the phrases:

'I understand how you feel' or *'I completely understand'*, or equivalent, as these are gifts for an angry patient: *'How can you understand unless you have got it!'*; *'Oh no you don't!'*

5.2.1.h. Reassuring the patient

Possible phrases you may use to reassure a patient are:

'I'm not worried about that.'

'Now, because this is important for you, it makes it important for me.'

'No, nothing is silly. We are trying to get to the bottom of this so that we can help you.'

'I think that's an absolutely/perfectly normal response in someone in your situation. Other people in your situation would feel the same way.'

'You did the right thing.'

'You did exactly the right thing.'

'You did the right thing coming today.'

'That's very good news.'

'I'm very pleased about that.'

'I think what you did was incredibly inspiring.'

'We all say things in the heat of the moment that we don't mean.'

5.2.1.i. Silence

Don't be afraid of using silence appropriately. Make good use of pauses and allow the patient to express their emotions, for example, by crying, before you move on.

A good technique to get a silent patient talking is by using reflection.

'It's as if you're finding this very difficult.'

'You seem to be finding it very difficult to describe how you feel.'

If the patient remains mute after using these empathetic statements, then say:

'Mr X, what's going through your mind?'

'Mr X, what are you thinking?'

'Are you ready to carry on?'

'What I need to do is find out what's bothering you and see how we can help you today.'

5.2.1.j. Summarising

Summarising the main points of information gathering gives confidence to the patient that you have been listening, shows them they have been heard, helps clarify what they have told you and gives them an opportunity to correct any misunderstandings.

'Just to kind of recap what you've said so far . . .'

'You mentioned you have had chest pain for 3 days, and it's worse when you cough. Have I got that right?'

Summarising is a particularly useful tool to clarify the individual's PC and also the agreed management plan. Summarising is also a useful strategy if you get stuck during history-taking. The process of saying out loud what the patient has told you is often enough to get your mind back on track.

This should be followed by giving the opportunity to the patient to add any more details:

'Is there anything else you wanted to mention?'

'Are there any other important things that you want to mention?'

Don't ask these questions at the end of the consultation, where you would have to reopen the interview to listen and enquire about any of the issues disclosed.

5.2.2. Information sharing and giving

The CSA assesses your ability to discuss a problem, and share management plans, where relevant, with the patient accurately and sensitively. You will be expected to communicate factually correct information in a simple and effective way within the emotional context of the clinical setting.

This section goes through the essential communication skills necessary to share your medical thoughts and ideas with the patient having made a working diagnosis and formed some options for management.

Time should be devoted in the consultation to explanations of the diagnosis, the causation of the patient's condition and the prognosis, as well as information concerning treatment and drug therapy. Marks are not only awarded for your clinical knowledge in the subject; additional marks will be awarded for your communication skills. The examiners will observe, assess and mark the spoken interaction between the candidate and the patient. The marking schedule gives credit for particular techniques used within a general approach while conveying information.

When imparting new knowledge, remember to consider strategies for maintaining optimal doctor–patient communication despite the need for information giving. Medical terminology or jargon describes medical content precisely, and therefore makes it possible to be specific when one medical practitioner converses with another. However, the same medical terms may cause your patients to become frustrated and confused if not accompanied by an explanation in lay terms. Sometimes, this is appropriate; for example, *'dermatologist, by which we mean "skin doctor"'/'cardiologist, in other words, "heart doctor"'/'oncologist, which is another term for "cancer doctor"'*. At other times, it may be better to avoid medical jargon altogether and phrase details simply and clearly in an appropriate non-technical language that the patients can understand. Patients are much more likely to understand *'You have had a stroke'*, than *'The CT scan has shown an ischaemic CVA (cardiovascular accident)'*. Either way, it is important to be sensitive to the amount and kinds of words you use with people from different social backgrounds and with different intellectual capacities.

If medical jargon is used, the role players used in the CSA are trained to ask, *'What's that, doctor?'*, *'What does that mean, doctor?'* or *'I'm sorry, I didn't understand that, doctor'*. This means that every time you use jargon you lose 30 seconds or so explaining what you meant, and if this happens a few times you may fall short of time.

The quantity and quality of information doctors give to their patients varies hugely. In general, doctors give sparse information to their patients, with most patients wanting their doctor to provide more information than they do. In the CSA, the amount of information given to the patient should be directed by the patient. If you have a large amount of information you wish to share with the patient, it goes without saying that it is a good idea to give some thought to planning the way you will present it.

5.2.2.a. Explaining a diagnosis
The CSA assesses your ability to share and discuss a problem with the patient simply, clearly and sensitively. You should be able to communicate a diagnosis accurately and effectively to the patient, where appropriate. A simple structure to share and discuss a diagnosis with the patient is provided on pages 98–103.

5.2.2.b. Sharing management plans
The CSA assesses your ability to negotiate and share a management plan with the patient simply, clearly and sensitively. You should be able to communicate a mutually agreed plan of action accurately and effectively to the patient, where appropriate. A simple structure to negotiate and share a management plan with the patient is provided on pages 106–110.

Chapter 6

A systematic template for structuring a consultation in 10 minutes

A GP without insight into what happens during the consultation, without at least a basic sense of how it is structured or the basic vocabulary to reflect on it, is not likely to be successful. In the CSA, you will be expected to demonstrate (to the examiner) proficiency in your ability to conduct effectively a well-focused, systematic and fluent 10-minute consultation. The primary aim of the book is to equip the reader with the underpinning knowledge, understanding, skills and attitude effectively required for successfully structuring a focused GP consultation in 10 minutes.

This chapter concentrates on issues of basic form and structure of a consultation. It brings you up to speed on how to perform an overall focused clinical assessment, establish a diagnosis and formulate a shared management plan competently within 10 minutes. It systematically guides you through the essential features of how to take an adequate medical history, conduct an appropriate clinical examination, formulate a list of possible differential diagnoses and negotiate a management plan, using your 10 minutes effectively, proficiently and preciously. Keeping to this consultation structure will ensure all domains of performance are covered appropriately within the allocated 10 minutes.

Furthermore, numerous examples of useful questions that could be asked of the patient to get to the crux of the problem, when to ask these questions, how to ask these questions sensitively, how to explain examinations correctly, how to communicate results/diagnosis and how to negotiate sensible management options with patients, in the right way, are all provided.

Presented following is a systematic, ordered, stepwise approach to structuring methodically a 10-minute focused consultation in the CSA. The overall shape and characteristics are that of the classic GP consultation. In other words, the patient will begin by doing most of the talking, with the doctor beginning to do more as the problem is explored, and with both parties negotiating together towards the end.

This purposeful, schematic and practical framework is not a chronologically ordered structure representing the elements of a consultation in the order in which they happen. Not all consultations will move exactly through these headings, and it is not intended to represent a sequential account (first this happens, then this . . .). Generally speaking, each consultation has its own momentum and requires a different approach tailored to the individual. Patients of differing age, class, gender, race and cultural and ethnic background have different needs and expectations and you should be able to adapt your consultation accordingly. Anything can affect the consultation structure and dynamics, and it helps to have a flexible, systematic and holistic consulting style. With experience, your own consulting style will change with the patient, but it is important to have some measure of consistency in approach to start with and have a framework that acts as a checklist if you are unsure where you are going.

It may not be possible to cover all of these headings within a single 10-minute consultation. Thinking about the key issues right from the start of the consultation will help you decide which areas to focus on during history-taking and examination as well as for management.

History

Several complaints are common in general practice, and the main elements of history-taking are described following in turn under the specific headings. It must be emphasised that these features that make up the complete medical history do not have to be addressed in any particular order, but their timing must seem appropriate and the consultation should have a sense of progress.

6.1. Introduction

6.2. Open consultation: presenting complaint (PC)

6.3. History of presenting complaint (HPC)

6.4. Red flags

6.5. Patient health beliefs, understanding and preferences: ideas, concerns and expectations (ICE)

6.6. Past medical history (PMH)/Past surgical history/Previous hospital admissions

6.7. Drug history (DH) and allergies

6.8. Family history (FH)

6.9. Psychosocial history (PSH)
   — If applicable: smoking, alcohol, illicit drugs, occupation, finances, driving, marital status/family structure/relationships/social networks, social setting/home situation, pets, major hobbies, ethnicity, culture and religion, effect of problem on patient's life/activities of daily living (ADL) and family, and mood and anxiety

The introduction and opening of the consultation should take about 1½ minutes. The main bulk of the consultation (HPC, red flags, ICE, relevant PMH, DH, FH and PSH) should take around 3–4 minutes to complete.

Examination

6.10. Physical examination

    6.10.1. Obtain informed consent and offer chaperone

    6.10.2. Perform targeted clinical examination

The physical examination should take a maximum of 2 minutes to perform.

Investigation

6.11. Results of investigations

Clinical management

6.12. Clinical management: diagnosis and management

    6.12.1. Diagnosis

        6.12.1.a. Inform diagnosis

        6.12.1.b. Explore patient's understanding of diagnosis

        6.12.1.c. Identify and explore patient's concerns about diagnosis

        6.12.1.d. Establish what and how much information patient would like

        6.12.1.e. Explain diagnosis: aetiology/pathophysiology, risk factors and triggers

        6.12.1.f. Seek feedback to check patient understanding

        6.12.1.g. Summarise

    6.12.2. Management

        6.12.2.a. Reassurance, if appropriate

        6.12.2.b. Explain things patient can do themselves: lifestyle advice

        6.12.2.c. Explain things you can offer patient: biopsychosocial

        6.12.2.d. Explain things patient may need to refrain from

        6.12.2.e. Further investigation, if appropriate

        6.12.2.f. Health promotion

        6.12.2.g. Seek feedback to check patient understanding

        6.12.2.h. Summarise

Clinical management (discussing the diagnosis and management) should take about 2–3 minutes to complete.

Ending the consultation

6.13. Summarise

6.14. Safety-net

6.15. Follow-up

6.16. Further information

6.17. Take responsibility for any gaps in understanding shown by the patient

6.18. Deal with any extra issues

6.19. Close consultation

Ending the consultation should take about 1 minute to complete.

Timing

It is important to split the 10 minutes (exactly 600 seconds) into a ratio between data gathering and clinical management so that all the time isn't spent in history-taking and there is enough time in the consultation for sharing management.

A useful structure for how to manage those all-important 10 minutes is:

- Introduction and opening of the consultation should take about 1½ minutes

- Main bulk of the consultation (HPC, red flags, ICE, relevant PMH, DH, FH and PSH) should take around 3–4 minutes to complete

- Targeted clinical examination should take a maximum of 2 minutes to perform

- Clinical management (formulating a diagnosis and management plan, and decision sharing) should take about 2–3 minutes

- Summarising, safety-netting, arranging follow-up, offering further information, taking responsibility for any gaps in understanding shown by the patient and closing the consultation should take about 1 minute to complete

Write down the following key steps of the focused clinical consultation at the beginning of the CSA:
- Introduction
- Open consultation: PC
- HPC
- Red flags
- Patient health beliefs, understanding and preferences: ICE
- PMH/Past surgical history/Previous hospital admissions
- DH and allergies
- FH
- PSH: smoking, alcohol, illicit drugs, occupation, finances, driving, marital status/family structure/relationships/social networks, social setting/home situation, pets, major hobbies, ethnicity, culture and religion, effect of problem on patient's life/ADL and family, and mood and anxiety
- Physical examination
- Explain diagnosis
- Share management
- End consultation: summarise, safety-net/follow-up, further information, take responsibility for any gaps in understanding shown by the patient, deal with any extra issues, close consultation

A quick glance at this checklist if you get stuck can be extremely useful to get you going again.

This can be abbreviated as follows.
- Intro
- PC
- HPC
- RF
- ICE
- PMH
- DH
- FH
- PSH
- Ex
- Dx
- Mx
- End Cx

The 10-minute CSA consultation

The buzzer will sound to mark the start of the CSA assessment, and the first patient will knock and enter your consulting room. Make a note of how old the patient is, if they are older or have a disability, open the door when they knock and help them to their chair.

6.1. Introduction

At the beginning of the consultation, stand up, smile, make eye contact and shake the patient's hand. Start with a good introduction (the opening greeting). Greet and welcome the patient politely into the consultation room, using their name:

> 'Hello, good morning, Mr/Mrs/Miss X. Please do take a seat.'
> (Show to the chair)

Introduce yourself to the patient (or surrogate parent/carer), using your professional title and surname:

> 'My name's Dr X. I'm a GP registrar.'

Try to establish rapport using phrases such as:

> 'Nice to meet you.'
> 'Pleased to meet you.'
> 'It's lovely to meet you.'
> 'We have not met before, have we? Well, it's lovely to meet you.'
> 'I can see you are new to the practice. Well, it's lovely to meet you.'

Other comments to help build a good rapport and connect with the patient include:

> 'I hope you have not had to wait too long in the waiting area.'
> 'I hope we have not kept you waiting too long, Mr X.'

If there is a second person with the patient, you should always find out the relationship between the two.

In summary, all consultations should begin with an opening greeting that sounds natural and fluent, such as:

'Hello, good morning Mr/Mrs/Miss X. Nice to meet you. Please do take a seat. My name's Dr X. I'm a GP registrar.'

6.2. Open consultation: presenting complaint (PC)

Open the consultation with open questions to identify the patient's agenda.

Use an open question at the start of a consultation to discover the reason(s) for the patient's attendance; that is, to identify the reason(s) for a patient's contact, their PC and concerns. Use an open question that you feel comfortable with and that sounds natural and caring:

'What can I do for you (today)?'
'How can I help you (today)?'
'Tell me, what seems to be the problem?'
'What prompted you to make the appointment today?'

Patient: *'I have a headache'* or *'I have a sore throat.'*

Respond with a caring statement:
'Oh, I'm sorry to hear that.'

Don't open the consultation with the open question:
'What brought you here (today)?'

Once you have identified the main reason(s) for the patient's visit, ask a second open question to allow the patient to elaborate on the presenting problem fully:

'Can you tell me a little bit more about that, please?'
'Can you say more/a little bit more about that, please?'
'Can you explain this to me in a bit more detail?'
'It would help me if I knew more about . . . (that).'
'Tell me more about . . .'
'And then . . .?'

Avoid interrupting patients before they have completed important statements about their complaint(s) and/or concern(s). The assessment of the patient should be done verbally and non-verbally. Listen actively (for up to a minute) to what the patient says and how they say it, and respond appropriately. Give the patient a chance to talk about what they want to freely, let them explain some of the things that are worrying them and encourage storytelling in their own words. Respond with genuine interest, and encourage the patient's contribution using various prompts (verbal and non-verbal), such as nodding your head, leaning forward, good eye contact or using expressions such as *'mmm'*, *'go on'*, *'sure'*, *'right'*, *'yes'*, *'good'* or some other emollient phrase.

If the patient uses jargon, for example 'funny turn', 'dizzy spell', 'dizziness', 'migraine', 'depression', 'anxious', 'paranoid', you need to seek clarification as to what exactly they mean.

> *'What do you mean by a "funny turn"/"dizzy spell"/"dizziness"?'*

> *'Oh, I'm sorry to hear that.'*
> *'Can you tell me a little bit more about that, please?'*

If a patient requests something specific, such as a particular medication, like the oral contraceptive pill (OCP), antibiotics, sleeping tablets or 'anti-stress pills', or a particular test, such as the prostate-specific antigen (PSA) test, candidates can often be taken by surprise. To deal with this, one should respond appropriately by saying:

> *'It would help me if I knew a little bit more about why you want the X?'*
> *'Tell me, what seems to be the problem?'*

> *'Oh, I'm sorry to hear that.'*
> *'Can you tell me a little bit more about that, please?'*

If you are ever stuck in the CSA, other useful open questions than can be used to facilitate the doctor–patient dialogue and elicit more information include:

> *'Tell me how it all started?'* or *'How did it all begin?'*
> *'How long has it been going on for?'*
> *'If you go back to the day it started, can you tell me exactly what happened?'*
> *'What was the first thing you noticed?'*

The introduction and opening of the consultation should take about 1½ minutes.

6.3. History of presenting complaint (HPC)

Moving on, assess the clinical problem by closing down in the assessment phase (HPC). Remember, the CSA is not a test of the ability to take a comprehensive history about the problem presented, but an assessment of the ability to perform a focused clinical assessment of the patient.

When closing down, it is sometimes helpful to warn the patient that you will be asking a set of brief and direct questions, which can help them focus. This can be done by using the suggested phrases:

'Is it okay if I ask you a few specific questions about your (symptom)?'

'I would like to ask you a few specific questions about your (symptom), if that's okay?'

'Would it be okay if I asked you some specific questions about your (symptom)?'

'Would it be okay if I asked you some specific questions now?'

'May I ask you a few specific questions about your (symptom), if that's okay?'

'I'm going to ask you some specific questions about your (symptom), if that's okay with you?'

Then take a history focused on the patient's PC with a series of closed questions. Closed questions effectively clinch and concentrate on further details of the clinical history and help take an efficient and factual account of the patient's problem. They should be used appropriately: primarily to assess the nature and duration/time course of any events, and then to define the pattern of symptoms to distinguish between mild and serious illness and explore diagnostic hypotheses. It makes sense to gather this clinical data bearing in mind the probabilities of underlying diseases.

The following features should be ascertained when assessing any PC, where appropriate:

◆ Nature (character)

◆ Onset

◆ Duration/Time course

◆ Frequency

◆ Trigger (precipitating) factors

◆ Exacerbating (aggravating) and relieving factors

◆ Severity and social disruption of illness

This can be done by asking the following list of suggested questions:

◆ Nature (character)
  'Describe the (symptom).'

◆ Onset
  'When did it start?'
  'How did it all begin?'
  'Did it start suddenly or gradually?'
  'If you go back to the day it started, can you tell me exactly what happened?'
  or *'What were you doing when it started?'* or *'Thinking about when it started, were you doing anything out of the ordinary or anything different?'*

◆ Duration/Time course
  'How long has it been going on for?'

◆ Frequency
  'Is the (symptom) there all the time, or does it come and go?'
  — If intermittent:
    'How often does it occur?'
    'How long does it last for?'
  'Does the (symptom) vary in intensity during the day?' or *'Is the (symptom) worse at any particular time of the day?'*
  'Is it getting better, worse or is it the same?'
  'Have you had anything like this in the past/before?' or *'Have you ever had this before?'*

◆ Trigger (precipitating) factors
  'What brings the (symptom) on?' or *'Does anything bring the (symptom) on?'*

◆ Exacerbating (aggravating) and relieving factors
  'What makes the (symptom) better?' or *'Does anything make the (symptom) better?'* or *'Is there anything you have found that makes the (symptom) better?'*
  'What makes the (symptom) worse?' or *'Does anything make the (symptom) worse?'* or *'Is there anything you have found that makes the (symptom) worse?'*

'Have you taken anything for the (symptom)?'

'What did you take?'

'How much X did you take?'

'Have you tried anything else for the (symptom)?'

'What other therapies have you tried?' (Physiotherapy, acupuncture, hypno-therapy, homeopathy, osteopathy, etc.)

◆ Severity and social disruption of illness

'How bad is the (symptom) on a scale of 0 to 10, 10 being the worst (symptom) you have ever had and 0 being no (symptom) at all?'

'Does the (symptom) interfere with your life/daily activities/day-to-day life?'

'How is the (symptom) affecting your life/daily activities/day-to-day life?'

'How is the (symptom) affecting the things you do at home, such as cooking, cleaning, shopping or do-it-yourself (DIY)?'

'Does the (symptom) stop you from doing anything?'

'Does the (symptom) stop you from sleeping?'

'Does the (symptom) disturb your sleep?'

'You mentioned that the (symptom) is affecting you in quite a lot of different ways. Can you tell me, in what different ways it is affecting you?'

'You mentioned that the (symptom) is stopping you from doing your job. Can I ask what that is?'

'How does your (symptom) affect your life as an X?' or *'How is this (symptom) affecting your job as an X?'*

'What changes have you had to make to your life because of the (symptom)?'

'Can you tell me who else is affected by the problem?'

Then define the pattern of symptoms to distinguish between mild and serious illness and explore diagnostic hypotheses; that is, enquire about associated symptoms and undertake a relevant general systems review. For example, if the patient presented with chest pain, you would enquire about the following pertinent symptoms from relevant system(s) to differentiate various possible diagnostic lines:

'Apart from the chest pain, how do you feel in yourself?'

'Is the chest pain accompanied by any other features?' (Nausea? Sweating? Shortness of breath?)

'Do you have a cough?'

'Do you cough anything up?' (Sputum)

'How much sputum do you cough up each day?' (A spoonful/egg-cupful/teacupful)

'What colour is the sputum?'

'Is the sputum bloodstained?' (Haemoptysis)

'Do you get short of breath?' (Dyspnoea)

'Is breathing more difficult when you lie flat?' (Orthopnoea)

'Do you wake up gasping for breath at night?' (Paroxysmal nocturnal dyspnoea)

'Have you had any palpitations?'

'Do your ankles swell?' (Peripheral oedema)

If appropriate, you may also enquire about relevant symptoms from other systems, such as the gastro-intestinal/digestive system.

The nature of follow-up questions should make sense and be appropriately based around previous responses so that the consultation follows a logical sequence and progresses easily. For example, if the patient complains of chest pain, *'I had some chest pain yesterday, doctor'*, your subsequent enquiry should explore the chest pain in a bit more detail: *'Can you tell me a little bit more about the chest pain, please?'* Don't ignore patient clues and start asking about the presence of a cough, shortness of breath or palpitations. Only once you have adequately explored the chest pain, should you ask about the presence or absence of symptoms to rule in and rule out relevant diagnoses.

HPC of pain

Pain is one of the commonest symptoms presented to doctors in medicine. It accounts for over 50% of consultations in general practice. Taking an adequate pain history is absolutely essential for accurately making a diagnosis of the pain. The salient points that need to be identified in any pain history include the specific features of the pain (site, onset, duration/time course and frequency), its characteristics (nature/character, radiation, triggers/precipitating factors, exacerbating and relieving factors, and associated symptoms) and the impact of the pain on ADL.

A good and simple framework is to use the SOCRATES acronym, which is an acronym for the headings:

- **S**ite

- **O**nset (duration and frequency)

- **C**haracter (nature)

- **R**adiation

- **A**ssociated symptoms (including relevant red flags and general systems review, where appropriate)

- **T**iming and **T**riggers (precipitating factors)

- **E**xacerbating (aggravating) and relieving factors

- **S**everity and **S**ocial disruption of pain

These can be ascertained using the following suggested questions:

- **S**ite
  'Where exactly is the pain?'

- **O**nset (duration and frequency)
  'When did the pain start?'
  'How did it all begin?'
  'Did it start suddenly or gradually?'
  'If you go back to the day it started, can you tell me exactly what happened?'
  or *'What were you doing when it started?'* or *'Thinking back to when it started, were you doing anything out of the ordinary or anything different?'*
  'How long has it been going on for?'
  'Is the pain there all the time, or does it come and go?'
  —If intermittent:
      'How often does it occur?'
      'How long does it last for?'
  'Is it getting better, worse or is it the same?'
  'Have you had anything like this in the past/before?' or *'Have you ever had this before?'*

◆ **C**haracter (nature)

'*Describe the pain.*'

'*Is it dull/aching/sharp/stabbing/knife-like/gripping/throbbing/burning/ crushing/heaviness/tightness/crampy/shooting?*'

◆ **R**adiation

'*Does the pain spread anywhere, or does it stay in the . . .?*'

◆ **A**ssociated symptoms (including relevant red flags and general systems review, where appropriate)

'*Apart from the pain, how do you feel in yourself?*'

'*Is the pain accompanied by any other features?*'

'*Do you have a . . .?*'

◆ **T**iming and **T**riggers (precipitating factors)

'*Does the pain vary in intensity during the day?*' or '*Is the pain worse at any particular time of the day?*'

'*What brings the pain on?*' or '*Does anything bring the pain on?*'

◆ **E**xacerbating (aggravating) and relieving factors

'*What makes the pain better?*' or '*Does anything make the pain better?*' or '*Is there anything you have found that makes the pain better?*'

'*What makes the pain worse?*' or '*Does anything make the pain worse?*' or '*Is there anything you have found that makes the pain worse?*'

'*Have you taken anything for the pain?*'

'*What painkillers did you take?*'

'*How much X did you take?*'

'*Have you tried anything else for the pain?*'

'*What other therapies have you tried?*' (Physiotherapy, acupuncture, hypno-therapy, homeopathy, osteopathy, etc.)

◆ **S**everity and **S**ocial disruption of pain

'*How bad is the pain on a scale of 0 to 10, 10 being the worst pain you have ever had and 0 being no pain at all?*'

'*Does the pain interfere with your life/daily activities/day-to-day life?*'

'*How is the pain affecting your life/daily activities/day-to-day life?*'

'*How is the pain affecting the things you do at home, such as cooking, cleaning, shopping or DIY?*'

'Does the pain stop you from doing anything?'

'Does the pain stop you from sleeping?'

'Does the pain disturb your sleep?'

'You mentioned that the pain is affecting you in quite a lot of different ways. Can you tell me, in what different ways it is affecting you?'

'You mentioned that the pain is stopping you from doing your job. Can I ask what that is?'

'How does your pain affect your life as an X?' or 'How is this pain affecting your job as an X?'

'What changes have you had to make to your life because of the pain?'

'Can you tell me who else is affected by the problem?'

6.4. Red flags

An important and relevant part of initial data gathering is to exclude serious organic pathology and emergency situations. Red flags, also known as alarm symptoms, are very unlikely to be known beforehand or offered spontaneously by the patient and have to be directly elicited. Red flags don't necessarily always need to be asked about, but relevant ones should be, when appropriate.

It is imperative that you take adequate steps to rule in or rule out any likely serious underlying disease, where appropriate. You should ask questions around relevant hypotheses (medical safety), taking into account the knowledge and understanding of epidemiology in the community. You need to be aware of what is likely, what is less likely and what is unlikely but relevant. Use your underlying medical knowledge in conjunction with what might be the likely prevalence, in terms of gender and age of the patient, when identifying red flags. You should not resort to asking about symptom lists; this is often more like a safe medical refuge (aimed at preventing errors in clinical practice) than garnering key clinical points.

For example, if an older patient presents with a history of intermittent rectal bleeding, appropriate red flags to identify in your clinical assessment would include:

◆ Nature of blood
  'Is the blood on the surface of the stool or on the paper or mixed with the stool?'

◆ Change in bowel habit
  'Have there been any changes in the character or frequency of your bowel movements?'

◆ Loss of appetite
  'Have there been any changes in your appetite?'

◆ Weight loss
  'Have there been any changes in your weight?'

The presence of red flags should raise concerns about bowel cancer.

Again, it may be helpful to warn the patient that you will be asking a set of direct questions to help them focus:

'In order to rule out/make sure this isn't a serious medical problem, I'd like to ask you a few specific questions.'

You may also find it useful to ask a more general open question first:

'Apart from the bleeding from your back passage, how do you feel in yourself?'

'Apart from the bleeding from your back passage, how do you feel in general terms?'

6.5. Patient health beliefs, understanding and preferences: ideas, concerns and expectations (ICE)

Exploring an individual's health beliefs about a problem not only provides you with higher-quality information but also helps adopt a patient-centred approach, and patients are more satisfied with the care they receive.

Further valuable information you would seek on history-taking includes asking about the patient's ideas (thoughts/perceptions/beliefs/perspectives), understanding and concerns (worries) about their main problem(s) and expectations about possible treatment(s). All the ICE questions are very good inviting questions that allow the patient to come forward and talk about other things.

Ideas

Discover the patient's ideas and perspectives about their main problem(s), if any. Possible questions you may use to find out and explore the patient's underlying ideas, beliefs and perceptions of their problem(s) are:

'What do you think this might be?'
'What do you think might be going on?'
'What do you think might be causing it?'
'What do you think might be causing your symptoms?'

'What did you think this might be?'
'What did you think might be going on?'
'What did you think might be causing it?'
'What did you think might be causing your symptoms?'

'Do you have any ideas about what this might be?'
'Do you have any ideas about what might be going on?'
'Do you have any ideas about what might be causing it?'
'Do you have any ideas about what might be causing your symptoms?'

'Have you had any thoughts as to what this might be?'
'Have you had any thoughts as to what might be going on?'
'Have you had any thoughts as to what might be causing it?'
'Have you had any thoughts as to what might be causing your symptoms?'

'In terms of the pain, have you had any thoughts as to what this might be?'
'In terms of the pain, have you had any thoughts as to what might be going on?'
'In terms of the pain, have you had any thoughts as to what might be causing it?'
'In terms of the pain, have you had any thoughts as to what might be causing your pain?'

'You say that you know that you have a spot on your X-ray. Do you have any ideas about what this might be?'
'You say that you know that you have a spot on your X-ray. Do you have any ideas about what might be going on?'

'You say that you know that you have a spot on your X-ray. Do you have any ideas about what might be causing it?'

'You say that you know that you have a spot on your X-ray. Do you have any ideas about what might be causing this spot?'

'What did you think was going on with you when you felt this lump?'
'Do you know why we sent you for that test?'
'Why do you want this X-ray really badly?'
'What do you think the X-ray will show?'
'Why do you want the antibiotics?'
'What do you think the antibiotics will do?'
'Have you talked to your friends or family? What do they think it is?'

For example, a 60-year-old man with a 2-week history of a sore throat seems to be very concerned and demands investigations.

If asked, *'In terms of the sore throat, have you had any thoughts as to what this might be?'*, one patient might answer 'tonsillitis' because his friend had recently been diagnosed with acute tonsillitis and another patient might answer 'throat cancer' because he is a heavy smoker.

Occasionally, if you ask the patient, you may get the answer, *'You're the doctor, you tell me!'*, but this should not deter you.

Concerns

Exploring and acknowledging the patient's main concerns (worries) are what patients remember most: whether you took their concerns on board. Find out what the patient is worried about and allow them to voice their concerns fully.

Possible questions you may use to elicit and explore concerns of patients are:

'Is there anything about what's going on that's particularly worrying you?'

'Is there anything about these symptoms that's particularly worrying you?'

'Is there anything in particular that you are concerned about?'

'You said/mentioned earlier on that you're worried about the pain. Is there anything about the pain that's particularly worrying you?'

'Is there anything about having this test that's particularly worrying you?'

'Is there anything about hearing this diagnosis that's particularly worrying you?'

'What would be your worst fear with these symptoms?'

'Are you worried that this might be something serious?'

'Are you worried that this might be anything in particular?'

Expectations

Find out what the patient expects from the doctor's appointment. Possible questions you may use to explore the patient's expectations are:

'What do you hope I will be able to help you with today?'

'Is there anything in particular you were hoping I could do for you today?'

'Is there anything in particular you would like us to help you with today?'

'Have you had any thoughts as to what I might be able to do for you today?'

'What were you hoping I would do for this condition?'

'Did you want something specific when you came here today?'

6.6. Past medical history (PMH)/Past surgical history/Previous hospital admissions

Enquire about general health, all previous significant illnesses, all previous operations and specific diagnosis of hypertension, myocardial infarction, stroke, asthma, diabetes mellitus (DM), arthritis, tuberculosis (TB), rheumatic fever, epilepsy, anxiety and depression, where relevant. Identify any co-morbidity that may affect the diagnosis and/or management.

Again, signal to the patient that you are about to do this by saying something like:

'I would like to ask you a few questions about your general health, if that's okay?'

General

Ask a general question first before you close down on the specific diseases.

'Have you suffered from any previous illnesses?'

Or

'I can see from your records that you have . . .'

All past medical disorders and surgical procedures should then be enquired about, including any hospital admissions, where appropriate.

Medical

'Have you ever been found to have high blood pressure (BP)?'
  'Have you ever had a heart attack or a stroke?'
  'Do you have asthma, DM or arthritis?'
  'Have you had TB or rheumatic fever?'
  'Have you ever suffered from epileptic seizures/fits?'
  'Have you suffered from anxiety or depression?'

Surgical

'Have you had any operations in the past?'

Hospital admissions

'Have you ever had any hospital admissions?'

If yes:

> *'When were you in hospital?'*
> *'Why were you in hospital?'*

Obstetric (where appropriate)

'Have you had any pregnancies?'

> *'Were there any complications during pregnancy like high BP, DM or pre-eclampsia?'*
> *'How did you give birth?'*
> *'Were there any complications during labour?'*

6.7. Drug history (DH) and allergies

Information about current prescription and non-prescription medication and doses that might be relevant, all allergic reactions (including any known reaction to antimicrobial agents) and adverse effects should be enquired about.

DH

'Do you take any medication?'

   'What medication do you take?'

   'Are you taking any OTC medication?'

   'Are you on the OCP?'

   'Are you on hormone replacement therapy?'

   'Do you take any herbal or homeopathic medicines/remedies or any health foods?'

Drug allergies

'Do you have any drug allergies?'

   'Are you allergic to X?'

Adverse drug reactions/Side effects

'Have any medicines ever upset you?'

   'How have they upset you?'

6.8. Family history (FH)

Ask if there are any problems that run in the family (significant illnesses in blood relatives), such as hypertension, DM or premature cardiovascular disease, and any FH of hereditary disorders, where relevant.

Again, signal to the patient that you are about to do this by saying something like:

'I would just like to ask you a few questions about your family, if that's okay?'

Then elicit relevant FH:

'Do any illnesses run in your family?'
'Do you have any brothers or sisters?'
'Are you father, mother, brother(s), sister(s) still alive?'

If still alive:

'Do they have any current illnesses?'

If they died:

'At what age did they pass away?'
'What did they die of?'

6.9. Psychosocial history (PSH)

Any modern account of the consultation begins with an understanding that each doctor–patient interview is likely to involve biomedical (physical), social and psychological factors. Sometimes, one of these areas will be emphasised more than the others, but it is essential to develop the necessary skills to identify and explore the relevant social and psychological aspects of the presentation to place the patient's problem in appropriate psychosocial contexts. You must interact with the patient in a manner that demonstrates an understanding of the social and psychological effects of the problem on the patient and their family, and vice versa. Exploring the social and psychological impact of the symptom(s) on the patient's daily life also helps you adopt a patient-centred approach.

Explore the relevant psychosocial aspects of the presentation to establish a complete picture of the patient's PC. Show that you understand the effect of the problem on the patient's life and their family. How does the symptom fit into the patient's social context? How is the problem affecting the patient's everyday life rather than just their health? What impact does the illness have on the patient's lifestyle, including work, home, family and leisure activities?

Social history

The following are common and important elements of the social history that should be ascertained, where appropriate:

- Smoking history
  - Current, ex-smoker or never smoked
  - Type of tobacco
  - Pack-year exposure
- Alcohol history
  - Alcohol consumption – current and previous, in units
- Illicit drugs/Recreational use of drugs
- Occupation
  - Employment/Unemployment
  - Present occupation
  - Full occupational history for appropriate medical conditions
- Finances
- Driving
- Marital status/Family structure/Relationships/Social networks
  - Health of partner or principal carer
  - Children
  - Extended family
  - Friends
- Social setting/Home situation
  - Type of accommodation
  - Access to essential amenities
- Pets
- Major hobbies
- Ethnicity, culture and religion
- Effect of problem on patient's life/ADL and family

How relevant these are will vary from case to case.

Don't launch straight into taking a social history without an introduction or gaining permission. It is sometimes helpful to explain to the patient exactly what you are going to do by saying something like:

'I would like to ask you a couple more things, if that's okay?'

Smoking

'Do you smoke?'

If yes:

'How many do you smoke a day?'

'How long have you been smoking?' or *'When did you start to smoke?'*

If no:

'Have you ever smoked?'

Alcohol

'Do you drink alcohol?'

If yes:

'How much do you drink?'

'How long have you been drinking that amount for?'

Illicit drugs/Recreational use of drugs

'Have you used any street drugs before?' or *'Have you ever used any non-prescription drugs?'*

If yes:

'What have you used?'

'When did you use them?'

'How long did you use them for?'

Occupation

'What do you do for a living?' or *'You mentioned that the (symptom) is stopping you from doing your job. Can I ask what that is?'*

'What does your job involve?'

'How are things at work?'

'Has anything happened at work?'

'How does your (symptom) affect your life as an X?' or *'How is this (symptom) affecting your job as an X?'*

'Have you spoken to anyone at work about your (symptom)?'

'Is there an occupational health department or health and safety officer you can consult at work?'

Finances

'Do you have any financial worries?'

Driving

'Do you drive?'

'How is the (symptom) affecting your ability to drive?'

Marital status/Family structure/Relationships/Social networks

'Who is at home with you?'

'Are you single, married, widowed or divorced?'

'Is your partner healthy?'

'How many children have you got?'

'Are your children healthy?'

'How are things at home?'

'Has anything happened at home?'

Social setting/Home situation

'What is your home like?'

'Do you have to manage stairs?'

'What facilities have you got at home?'

'Do you have any carers?'

'Do you have meals on wheels?'

Pets

'Do you have any pets?'

Major hobbies

'What are your interests and hobbies?'

   'How do you spend your free time?'

   'Aside from work, what keeps you busy?'

   'What do you enjoy spending your time doing?'

Ethnicity, culture and religion

'How would you describe your ethnicity/culture?'

   'Do you follow a religion?'

Effect of problem on patient's life/ADL and family

'Does the (symptom)/it interfere with your life/daily activities/day-to-day life?'

   'How is the (symptom)/it affecting your life/daily activities/day-to-day life?'

   'How is the (symptom)/it affecting the things you do at home, such as cooking, cleaning, shopping or DIY?'

   'Does the (symptom)/it stop you from doing anything?'

   'Does the (symptom)/it stop you from sleeping?'

   'Does the (symptom)/it disturb your sleep?'

   'You mentioned that the (symptom)/it is affecting you in quite a lot of different ways. Can you tell me, in what different ways it is affecting you?'

   'What changes have you had to make to your life because of this problem?'

   'Can you tell me who else is affected by the problem?'

Psychological history

The following areas of the psychological history should be ascertained, where appropriate:

♦ Depression

♦ Anxiety

Assessing depression

Presented following is a useful tool that can be used by GPs in identifying patients with a depressive illness and to formally assess depression.

Remember that sensitive information should be asked for in a different manner to routine medical symptoms. Signposting to the patient that one is entering a potentially difficult territory is useful:

'I would like to ask you a few personal questions, if that's okay?'

'As it's relevant and may be important, I'd like to ask some sensitive questions, if that's okay?'

Start by asking a more general open question first:

'How are you feeling at the moment?' or

'How do you feel within yourself?'

'Oh, I'm sorry to hear that.'

'Can you tell me a little bit more about that, please?'

Then assess the core characteristic features of depression:

♦ Low mood

♦ Anhedonia (loss/lack of interest, enjoyment or pleasure)

♦ Anergia (loss/lack of energy)

Low mood

'During the last month, have you been feeling particularly down/low, depressed or hopeless?'

'I would like to know if there have been any times during the last month when you have been feeling particularly down/low, depressed or hopeless?'

'I would like to know if there have been any times when you have felt particularly down/low, depressed or hopeless?'

Anhedonia

'During the last month, have you lost interest, enjoyment or pleasure in doing things?'

'During the last month, have you often been bothered by having little interest, enjoyment or pleasure in doing things?'

'Do you still enjoy the things you used to enjoy doing?'

'Is there anything that you are able to get enjoyment out of?'

Anergia

'During the last month, have you often been bothered by feeling tired or had little energy?'

If appropriate, enquire about any secondary/accessory (biological and cognitive) symptoms of depression, such as reduced concentration and attention, reduced self-esteem and self-confidence, feelings of worthlessness or guilt, disturbed sleep, loss of interest in sex (loss of libido), diminished appetite and weight loss, to establish the severity of the patient's depression.

Reduced concentration and attention

'During the last month, have you often been bothered by poor concentration?'

'During the last month, have you often been bothered by trouble concentrating on things, such as reading the newspaper or watching television?'

Reduced self-esteem and self-confidence

'During the last month, have you often been bothered by low self-esteem and self-confidence?'

Feelings of worthlessness or guilt

'During the last month, have you often been bothered by feelings of worthlessness or guilt?'

Disturbed sleep

'During the last month, have you often been bothered by trouble falling or staying asleep, or sleeping too much?'

Loss of interest in sex

'During the last month, have you often been bothered by loss of interest in sex?'

Diminished appetite

'During the last month, have you often been bothered by poor appetite or overeating?'
   'Have there been any changes in your appetite?'
   'How's your appetite?'

Weight loss

'Have there been any changes in your weight?'

You may need to make a risk assessment depending on what the depression screening reveals (*see* 7.5.). Asking about suicidal feelings fits very nicely with asking about mood disturbance.

Note: NICE recommends that any patient who may have depression (especially those with a past history of depression or who suffer from a chronic physical illness associated with functional impairment) should be asked the following two questions:

   'During the last month, have you been feeling down/low, depressed or hopeless?'
   'During the last month, have you often been bothered by having little interest or pleasure in doing things?'

If patients with a chronic physical health problem answer 'yes' to either question, the following three further questions should be asked to establish the severity of depression:

   'During the last month, have you often been bothered by feelings of worthlessness?'
   'During the last month, have you often been bothered by poor concentration?'
   'During the last month, have you often been bothered by thoughts of death?'[3]

Assessing anxiety

This is a useful tool that can be used in identifying patients with anxiety.

Again, signpost to the patient that one is entering a potentially sensitive area:

'I would like to ask you a few personal questions, if that's okay?'

'As it's relevant and may be important, I'd like to ask some sensitive questions, if that's okay?'

Start by asking a more general open question first:

'How are you feeling at the moment?' or

'How do you feel within yourself?'

'Oh, I'm sorry to hear that.'

'Can you tell me a little bit more about that, please?'

Then assess for anxiety using the following questions:

'Do you get anxious or agitated?'

'Do you feel tense or "wound up"?'

'Do you get a sort of frightened feeling, as if something awful is about to happen?'

'Do worrying thoughts go through your mind?'

'Can you sit at ease and feel relaxed?'

'Do you get a sort of frightened feeling, like "butterflies" in your stomach?'

'Do you feel restless, as if you have to be on the move?'

'Do you get sudden feelings of panic?'

Apart from the first question, the remaining seven questions have been taken from the hospital anxiety and depression questionnaire/scale used to determine the level of anxiety and depression that a patient is experiencing.[4]

The main bulk of the consultation (HPC, red flags, ICE, relevant PMH, DH, FH and PSH) should take around 3–4 minutes to complete.

6.10. Physical examination

Physical examination is another crucial milestone of data gathering. One reason a physical examination is carried out is to gather more relevant data for clinical judgement and choice of investigations. Secondly, it is performed to demonstrate proficiency in a clinical examination skill, an examination technique or the appropriate use of medical diagnostic equipment, accordingly.

After a history has been taken from the patient, if you decide that a physical examination forms an integral part of your focused clinical assessment of the case, you should decide on the appropriate clinical examination and then examine the patient, and your strategy and technique will be marked accordingly.

6.10.1. Obtain informed consent and offer chaperone

The examination must always be done after seeking appropriate consent, explaining to the patient what you are proposing to do in an examination and why you are doing it, and a chaperone must be offered, if necessary.

Ask permission before examining a patient:

'Is it okay if I examine you?'

Offer a chaperone, where appropriate:

'Would you like a chaperone?'

6.10.2. Perform targeted clinical examination

You should decide on a choice of relevant physical examination, explain to the patient what you want to examine (*see* examples on pages 95–96) and then skilfully perform a targeted examination in a rational sequence, giving the impression that you are competent and confident in the skills and techniques being assessed.

During your focused clinical examination of the patient, respect their dignity, show them courtesy and use skills that aid rapport building.

'I can see that you are struggling, Mr X.'

'I can see that you are in quite a lot of pain, Mr X.'

'I can see that you are quite breathless, Mr X.'

'Oh, I'm sorry about that.'

'If it's uncomfortable, please let me know.'

Once you have finished examining the patient, thank them:

'Okay then, Mr X, thank you for letting me have a look.'

Assist them in getting off the examination couch, getting dressed and so forth, if you feel help is needed. Don't forget to wash your hands or use the alcohol hand gel provided on the desk in your consulting room.

6.10.3. Examples

A few examples of focused clinical examinations you may be required to explain to patients in the CSA as part of your data gathering, such as the assessment of the upper respiratory tract, cerebellar system or measurement of a peak flow, are presented following. Simple suggestions offering straightforward explanations for carrying out these examinations are also provided.

Upper respiratory tract

'What I would like to do is check your temperature, feel your pulse, look at the back of your throat and inside your ears, and feel your neck to see if there are any swellings. Is that okay?'

'I'm really sorry. It does look quite bad.'

'Okay then, Mr X, thank you for letting me have a look.'

If the patient asks:

'Why do you want to check my temperature?'

Respond appropriately by saying:

'The reason I would like to check your temperature is that sometimes if an infection is causing the problem and one of the clues we get is that the body temperature goes up.'

Auroscope/Otoscope

'I'm going to have a look inside the good ear first to give me a comparison of what's normal for you. If it's uncomfortable, let me know.'

Tip: Get the biggest earpiece that goes comfortably into the patient's ear.

Peak expiratory flow rate

Explain the test first, demonstrate it yourself and then get the patient to do it.

'You have to do it standing up, the meter has to be set to zero each time, don't cover the shooting bit and hold it horizontal/flat to the floor (to avoid the effect of gravity). Breathe in, tight seal around the mouthpiece, and then breathe out as hard and as fast as you can, like you're blowing out a candle. We do this three times and we take the best reading. We then compare it to the expected peak flow for your height. You may feel a bit light-headed.'

Cerebellar signs

Dysdiadokinesia: rapid hand-turn test

'Palms up towards the ceiling. Touch your left palm with your right palm. Then take your right hand and put the palm up to the ceiling, and now keep doing that.'

'Now, do that with the other side.'

Dysmetria

This is tested using the point-to-point test in two different ways: the shin–heel test or the finger–nose test. In the exam, just carry out one of the point-to-point tests to assess for dysmetria. The shin–heel test is really difficult to explain; the finger–nose test is a lot easier. Ensure your instructions are clear and precise to avoid any confusion:

'Can I ask you to take the tip of your index finger of your right hand and touch it to the tip of your nose? Now, take that finger and touch it to the tip of my finger and back to your nose, now back to my finger, back to your nose, back to my finger and back to your nose.'

'Now, do that with the other side.'

Make them stretch, looking for intention tremor and pass pointing.

Practise focused physical examinations that are most likely to be tested in the CSA until you can explain and perform them confidently and smoothly.

Note: Sometimes, after performing an examination, you may need to ask a few more questions to come up with a sensible differential or accurate working diagnosis.

The clinical examination should take a maximum of 2 minutes to perform.

6.11. Results of investigations

Check the results of any investigations provided in the 'patient notes' before the patient enters your consulting room, as you may find some of this information useful within the consultation. You should integrate findings from the focused clinical assessment of the patient with additional information from the patient 'clinical records' for better clinical judgement.

6.12. Clinical management: diagnosis and management

6.12.1. Diagnosis

The CSA assesses your ability to establish an appropriate working diagnosis or construct a limited list of possible differential diagnoses reflecting the information gathered (during data gathering) using your clinical diagnostic skills. It is also designed to test your ability to share and discuss a diagnosis with the patient simply, clearly and sensitively.

You should be able to use relevant information obtained during data gathering to draw appropriate conclusions, establish a specific diagnosis or range of diagnoses and communicate this information accurately and effectively to the patient.

Establish diagnosis/differential diagnoses

You are expected to make an appropriate diagnosis/differential diagnoses that most likely fit(s) with the clinical history, examination and investigations you have gathered during the clinical assessment phase of the consultation.

You should consider the information gathered carefully and identify the key issues, which should be addressed in terms of the possible causes of the presentation. A likely, working diagnosis needs to be made or a sensible differential diagnoses list constructed, so that appropriate and adequate clinical decisions can be subsequently made. Common and serious medical conditions should be considered in the differential diagnoses.

Explain diagnosis

Having established a working diagnosis or constructed a limited list of possible differential diagnoses, this should be explained to the patient in a clear, concise, effective and confident manner in the patient's language. You will need to select the most appropriate information to communicate; tailor information to what the patient wants to know; provide information that is correct; explain issues in an appropriate way, avoiding medical jargon as much as possible; and respond and adapt to the emotional context of the consultation.

There are many ways in which a diagnosis may be imparted to the patient, some better than others, and following is a simple structure to act as a checklist – useful if you get stuck!

Points to consider in your discussion include:

6.12.1.a. Inform diagnosis

6.12.1.b. Explore patient's understanding of diagnosis

6.12.1.c. Identify and explore patient's concerns about diagnosis

6.12.1.d. Establish what and how much information patient would like

6.12.1.e. Explain diagnosis: aetiology/pathophysiology, risk factors and triggers

6.12.1.f. Seek feedback to check patient understanding

6.12.1.g. Summarise

6.12.1.a. Inform diagnosis

Enquiring about the patient's health beliefs (during data gathering) and incorporating these into your explanations later (during clinical management) is an important part of the work of general practice and is assessed within the interpersonal skills domain of the marking schedules used in the CSA.

Tell the patient about the likely diagnosis or possible differential diagnoses. The description of the diagnosis should be precise and tailored to the patient's level of comprehension and vocabulary, remembering that explanations are often most effective when you affirm a patient's health beliefs.

'From everything/what you have said, mentioned and described, and from examining you today, Mr X, there are a couple of things this could be. You mentioned earlier that you were worried about X. I don't think this is X, which I'm very pleased about. The most likely thing is something called ...'

Or

'From everything/what you have said, mentioned and described, and from examining you today, Mr X, there are a couple of things this could be. You mentioned earlier that you thought this may be due to X. Like you, I think the (symptom) might also be due to a ... trapped nerve ...'

Or

'There are a couple of things this could be. But I think the most likely thing is something called ...'

Elicit the patient's reactions to the information given and show empathy towards this:

'I'm sorry to have to tell you that.'

'I can see that you are upset hearing this news.'

'I can see that this has come as an awful shock/surprise to you.'

'I can see this has clearly upset you.'

'I can see that this seems to have made you very upset/sad/angry . . .'

6.12.1.b. Explore patient's understanding of diagnosis

When imparting clinical information, the patient's level of knowledge and understanding of medical and health matters should be established and your explanation should be appropriately adjusted to these.

'Can you tell me, is this something you have heard of before?'

'Have you heard of that before?'

'Does that mean anything to you?'

'How does that come across to you?'

'Tell me what you understand by that?'

'What does the term "angina" mean to you?'

'What do you know about having . . . high cholesterol . . . ?'

'Do you have any friends or family with X?'

6.12.1.c. Identify and explore patient's concerns about diagnosis

Show a particular ability to explore the individual's main concerns about the problem.

'Is there anything about hearing this diagnosis that's particularly worrying you?'

'Is there anything about what's going on that's particularly worrying you?'

6.12.1.d. Establish what and how much information patient would like

Ask patients what information they would like, and prioritise their information needs so that important needs can be dealt with first if time is short. Find out how much information the patient wants to know. Some patients prefer to know every little detail about what is going on, whereas others just like to know the basics at the moment.

'I would just like to ask, how much detail you would like me to go into?'

'What I mean is that some people prefer to know all the details about what is going on, whereas others just like to know the basics. How do you feel?'

'Are you the kind of person who prefers to know all the details about what is going on?'

'How much information would you like me to give you about your diagnosis?'

'Some people like to know everything all in one go, whereas others prefer to go little by little. How do you feel?'

6.12.1.e. Explain diagnosis: aetiology/pathophysiology, risk factors and triggers

The CSA is not a test of the amount of information conveyed during information sharing. A short explanation about the findings and problem may be enough, but it must be relevant, understandable and tuned to the patient in an appropriate language, without the use of jargon or inappropriate technical descriptions that patients do not understand.

Clearly explain the diagnosis to the patient, focusing on aetiology/pathophysiology, risk factors and triggers, and try to use the same words as the patient, if possible.

'Would you like me to go over some details with you?' or *'Would you like me to tell you a bit more about it?'* or *'I'll just go over some of the detail with you, if that's okay?'*

'Let's take this one step at a time, shall we?'

Aetiology/Pathophysiology

'Essentially, what happens is . . .'

Risk factors

'Anybody can get this, but there are some people who are more likely to get it than others. It is more common in people who smoke, drink, are overweight . . .'

Triggers

'Some of the things that could actually set it off are . . .'

6.12.1.f. Seek feedback to check patient understanding

When it comes to imparting new information and meaning to your patient, success can be measured by the extent to which your patient has understood what they have been told, and in order to be aware of this you need to actively seek feedback. This is a skill that should be in operation throughout your consultation. Aside from listening to what your patient actually says, you can be constantly aware of non-verbal signals. You can be aware of facial expressions, which may show puzzlement, confusion or lack of interest. You can become alert to frowns, raised eyebrows, blushes and blank looks. However, it is usually not possible to rely on this as your only means of feedback, so you need to become habituated to inviting the patient to ask questions on any aspect of the consultation they feel requires further clarification in order to check that they are with you at every stage. It is usually not enough to deliver all your information and then ask, *'Have you got any questions?'* Rather, it is better to get into the habit of checking with your patient after every new piece of information is given before moving on.

Possible prompts you may use to check for patient understanding before moving on are:

'How does that come across to you?'

'Does that mean anything to you?'

'Tell me what you understand by that.'

Always ask if they would like you to go over anything, and offer them a chance to ask questions:

'Is there anything you would like me to go over again?'

'Is there anything that you want me to explain again?'

'Do you want to ask me anything about that?'

You can also take responsibility for any gaps in understanding shown by the patient in response, in order to spare their anxiety over appearing slow or stupid, using phrases like:

'I'm not sure I explained that very well. Let me put it another way . . .'

'I am not sure that I explained that very well. Is there anything you would like me to go over again?'

'Is there anything I have said that I have not been clear about?'

'Is there anything about what I've just said that I wasn't clear about?'
'Is there anything I haven't explained clearly?'

The question *'What are you going to tell your husband/wife when you get home today?'* is the right question to ask only when you have identified that the patient's husband/wife has a particular concern about their health.

6.12.1.g. Summarise

Summarise the main points you want the patient to remember:

'I know it's a lot to take in, but just to summarise/recap, the key/main/important points that I want you to remember are . . .'

An example using asthma is provided following to practically illustrate this simple structure for explaining a diagnosis to the patient.

Inform diagnosis

'From everything you have said, mentioned and described, and from examining you today, Mr X, there are a couple of things this could be. You mentioned earlier that you were worried about . . . lung cancer/TB. I don't think this is lung cancer/TB, which I'm very pleased about. The most likely thing is something called asthma.'

'I'm sorry to have to tell you that.'

Explore patient's understanding of diagnosis

'Can you tell me, is this something you have heard of before?'

'What do you know about having asthma?'

Identify and explore patient's concerns about diagnosis

'Is there anything about hearing this diagnosis that's particularly worrying you?'

Establish what and how much information patient would like

'Would you like me to go over some details with you?'

'I would just like to ask, how much detail would you like me to go into?'

Explain diagnosis: aetiology/pathophysiology, risk factors and triggers

'Let's take this one step at a time, shall we?'

'When you breathe in, air goes in through your mouth, through your windpipe and through some breathing tubes into your lungs. Essentially, what happens in asthma is your breathing tubes become a bit narrow. That's when your chest becomes tight and wheezy and you can't breathe as easily.'

'Anybody can get this, but there are some people who are more likely to get it than others. It is more common in people who smoke, have eczema or hay fever and in those who have a family member with asthma.'

'Some of the things that could actually set it off are cold weather, exercise, pet hairs, smoke, dust and infections.'

'When people have asthma, sometimes they are fine, other times they find that *their chest is tight and wheezy and they struggle to breathe. What happens is your breathing tubes become a bit narrow. We call that an asthma attack.'*

   'What sets that off is different for different people.'

   ('What the blue inhaler does is open up the breathing tubes, making the breathing easier and better.')

Note: Avoid the use of medical jargon/euphemisms like 'allergen' or 'trigger', which some patients do not understand; instead, use the phrase *'sets it off'*.

Seek feedback to check patient understanding

'How does that come across to you?'

   'Is there anything you would like me to go over again?'

   'Do you want to ask me anything about that?'

Summarise

'I know it's a lot to take in, but just to summarise, the important points that I want you to remember are . . .'

6.12.2. Management

The CSA assesses your ability to devise a safe, shared and acceptable management plan to deal with the patient's problem(s), reflecting a deeper working knowledge underpinning current British best practice. It is also designed to test your ability to negotiate and share a management plan with the patient simply, clearly and sensitively.

You will be expected to formulate a plan of action, appropriate to the findings, in collaboration with the patient, and communicate this to the patient accurately and effectively.

Negotiate and share management plan

Guide the patient through the appropriate and sensible management options for their presentation, making them aware of the relative risks and benefits of the different approaches and involving them in decision-making.

The management methods employed should be safe and congruent with current accepted British general practice. Use the biopsychosocial model when planning management, firstly offering the things that the patient can do themselves to manage their symptoms, and secondly the things that you can offer. Remember, you may need to advise the person about the sort of things they should refrain from if their problem/diagnosis is likely to render them a source of danger to themselves or others.

Communication skills make an appreciable difference to clinical management. Again, there are many ways in which management can be shared with the patient, and provided following is a simple structure to act as a checklist – useful if you get stuck!

Points to consider in your discussion include:

6.12.2.a. Reassurance, if appropriate

6.12.2.b. Explain things patient can do themselves: lifestyle advice

6.12.2.c. Explain things you can offer patient: biopsychosocial

6.12.2.d. Explain things patient may need to refrain from

6.12.2.e. Further investigation, if appropriate

6.12.2.f. Health promotion

6.12.2.g. Seek feedback to check patient understanding

6.12.2.h. Summarise

6.12.2.a. Reassurance, if appropriate

'In terms of what we can do about it, the good news is that it is something we can usually treat quite well in general practice and hopefully settle it down.'
    'The good news is that it is something we can usually treat quite well.'

'There are lots of/various ways we could try to help you deal with this.'
'There are lots of/various ways we could help you approach this.'
'There are lots of/various ways we can try to help you.'

'There are lots of/various things we can do to try to help you deal with this.'
'There are lots of/various things we can do to help you approach this.'
'There are lots of/various things we can do to try to help you.'

'There are a couple of ways we could try to help you deal with this.'
'There are a couple of ways we could help you approach this.'
'There are a couple of ways we could try to help you.'

'There are things that you can do yourself and things that we can offer.'

6.12.2.b. Explain things patient can do themselves: lifestyle advice

Give relevant advice about lifestyle modifications/preventative management.
    'Things you can try to do yourself are cut back on your alcohol, stop smoking, exercise, lose some weight, take regular breaks at work, ask other colleagues to help when you're busy to relieve some stress and eat lots of fruit and vegetables.'
    'These are some of the things you can do to reduce the likelihood of these symptoms.'
    'What do you think about this?'

6.12.2.c. Explain things you can offer patient: biopsychosocial

The use of jargon should be avoided as much as possible, and details should be phrased simply and clearly in an appropriate non-technical language that the patient can understand. The pros and cons of different treatments should be discussed.
    'Things that we can offer are a specific type of medication, something called . . .'

'Can you tell me, is this something you have heard of before?'

'I'll just go over some of the details with you, if that's okay?'

'Essentially, what this tablet does is . . .'

'Hopefully the . . . (pain/swelling) will start to settle down in a few days.'

'However, there are side effects from the treatment, the most common being . . .'

'The other treatment option includes . . . physiotherapy/seeing a counsellor/ seeing a dietician/referral to a specialist . . .'

'What do you think about these options?'

'What I'm going to do is give you a prescription for . . . You should take one tablet X times day with/after food/on an empty stomach.'

6.12.2.d. Explain things patient may need to refrain from

You may need to give the patient relevant advice or instructions about the things they should refrain from if their problem/diagnosis may put them or others at risk of danger or harm, for example, driving, cycling, swimming, climbing ladders/ scaffoldings and work.

'I'm going to tell you something quite difficult now.'

'Unfortunately, because you have had . . . (an epileptic fit) . . ., I hope you will understand that you must not do anything which if you have a . . . (fit) . . . will put yourself or other people at danger.'

'What this means is that one of the things you won't be able to do is . . . (drive) anymore for . . . (1 year . . . the time being).'

'I'm sorry to have to tell you that.'

'How do you feel about that?'

6.12.2.e. Further investigation, if appropriate

Give rationale for any investigations, where appropriate.

'What we are going to have to do is arrange for some further tests to find out . . .'

'How do you feel about that?'

'Depending on what we find, you may need to have . . . further tests, some medicine(s) or see a specialist.'

'If there is anything else, then we will discuss that once we have the results because we don't know what's going on at the moment.'

6.12.2.f. Health promotion

Try to use opportunities in every consultation to promote good health. This should not just be a 'box-ticking' exercise but should be done where relevant by linking it to what the patient came in for. For instance, if a patient has a lower respiratory tract infection, then relevant, opportunistic health promotion would be to encourage smoking cessation.

'Did you know that smoking makes it more likely to get these infections and it makes it more difficult for your body to fight it on its own? Antibiotics will help this time. If you were ever thinking of cutting back, we can offer help.'

Don't just give very brief lifestyle advice (smoking, alcohol, diet, exercise, eating patterns, stress, etc.) at the end of every consultation in order to 'tick the box', unless deemed appropriate.

6.12.2.g. Seek feedback to check patient understanding

Check that the patient has understood before moving on, by asking:

'How does that come across to you?'

'Does that mean anything to you?'

'Tell me what you understand by that?'

Always ask if they would like you to go over anything, and offer them a chance to ask questions:

'Is there anything you would like me to go over again?'

'Is there anything that you want me to explain again?'

'Do you want to ask me anything about that?'

You can also take responsibility for any gaps in understanding shown by the patient in response, in order to spare their anxiety over appearing slow or stupid, using phrases like:

'I'm not sure I explained that very well. Let me put it another way . . .'

'I am not sure that I explained that very well. Is there anything you would like me to go over again?'

'Is there anything I have said that I have not been clear about?'

'Is there anything about what I've just said that I wasn't clear about?'

'Is there anything I haven't explained clearly?'

6.12.2.h. Summarise

Summarise the main points you want the patient to remember:

'I know it's a lot to take in, but just to summarise/recap, the key/main/important points that I want you to remember are . . .'

An example using gout is provided following to practically illustrate this simple structure for sharing management options with the patient.

Reassurance, if appropriate

'In terms of what we can do about it, the good news is that it is something we can usually treat quite well in general practice and hopefully settle it down.'

'There are lots of ways we could try to help you deal with this.'

'There are things that you can do yourself and things that we can offer.'

Explain things patient can do themselves: lifestyle advice

'Things you can try to do yourself are cut back on your alcohol and on certain foods, such as oily fish, mussels, sardines, mackerel, kidney, liver, red meat, beans and spinach.'

'These are some of the things you can do to reduce the likelihood of an attack.'

'What do you think about this?'

Explain things you can offer patient: biopsychosocial

'Things that we can offer include a specific type of medication, something called . . . (ibuprofen).' (Or any other non-steroidal anti-inflammatory drug)

'Can you tell me, is this something you have heard of before?'

'I'll just go over some of the details with you, if that's okay?'

'Essentially, this tablet not only helps with pain but will also start to work on the swelling.'

'But there are some people who cannot take this type of medication. So I would just like to ask you if you have problems with your stomach, such as indigestion or heartburn, or if you have asthma, because this tablet can set them off and that's why I ask.'

'So these are some of the groups of people who cannot take this type of painkiller.'

'What I'm going to do is give you a prescription for ibuprofen. You should take one tablet three times a day. It is really important that you take it with or just after a meal, as it can upset your stomach. I would like you to take it for the next few days. It should start helping with the pain really within the first day, and it should start helping with the swelling really within 2 or 3 days.'

Further investigation, if appropriate

'As we have discussed, essentially, what happens in gout is you get too much of a certain type of acid (called uric acid/urate) building up in your body. Two weeks after an attack has settled, we usually measure the level of this acid in your blood. We don't test the level during an attack because it tends to decrease/may be normal.'

Health promotion

'Did you know that losing weight, limiting/reducing alcohol consumption/intake, avoiding dehydration and exercise can all reduce the likelihood of an attack?'

Seek feedback to check patient understanding

'How does that come across to you?'

   'Is there anything you would like me to go over again?'

   'Do you want to ask me anything about that?'

Summarise

'I know it's a lot to take in, but just to summarise, the important points that I want you to remember are ...'

Clinical management skills should take about 2–3 minutes. This leaves around 1 minute for rounding up and ending the consultation: summarising, safety-netting, arranging follow-up, offering further information, taking responsibility for any gaps in understanding shown by the patient and closing the consultation with a definitive end.

6.13. Summarise

There should be a shared understanding before the patient leaves your consulting room. This can be confirmed by asking the patient to summarise what they have understood towards the end of the interview.

'You mentioned you have a wife/husband. What will you tell her/him when you get home?'

'Which bits of our chat have reassured you?'

'From our discussion, what will you take away with you?'

'Just so we know we're on the same page, what's our way forward from here?'

If it's a child and you want to reinforce something to the mother, you can sometimes quiz the child; for example, for chloramphenicol eye drops:

'Okay, so how often do you need to use these drops for the first 2 days? Then after that, how many times a day? Then how many days do you use it for? Until it's better, then how many extra days? Good lad.'

Alternatively, summarise the key take-home messages you want the patient to remember:

'I know it's a lot to take in, but just to summarise/recap, the key/main/important points that I want you to remember are . . .'

'I know it's a lot to take in, but I want you to remember that . . .'

6.14. Safety-net

Remember to safety-net appropriately and fully, and understand the significance of doing so. Effective safety-netting ensures a contingency plan has been well-defined to handle the worst-case clinical scenario.

You should give clear and specific advice to the patient about what to do if symptoms get worse or develop in some way that is unexpected, including a description of where and how to seek help, at any time of day or night.

'I'd expect your sore throat to last about a week, your congested nose to settle after about 1½ weeks and your cough to last 2–3 weeks, which may trouble you more at night. But if you run any further temperatures, or if you're short of breath in any way, or not getting better as I described, then please come back and see me.'

'If it's not changed at all in a couple of days and certainly if it gets worse, I would like you to come back and see me, so I can have a look at it again.'

'Please call back/come back to see me if you are at all worried/concerned.'

'I'd be happy to see your child at short notice.'

6.15. Follow-up

A consultation should not be seen as an isolated incident but rather as part of the continuum of the course of an illness. Make adequate arrangements for follow-up of patients that reflect the natural history of the problem with either yourself or another healthcare professional, for example, a nurse or a specialist.

For instance, if making a definite time for the next appointment:

'I would like you to come back and see me in . . ., if that's okay?'

'I would like you to see the nurse for a BP check in . . . 1 month.'

'Please book for a BP review in . . . 1 month with the nurse.'

You can also specify conditions and interval for follow-up:

'If you are not getting better in 4–6 weeks, I would like to see you again.'

6.16. Further information

Reinforce your explanations on diagnosis, management, safety-netting, etc. with written information, when appropriate.

Offer the patient additional, often more detailed information through a relevant PIL to take away and read, or ask them if they have access to the Internet and provide them with details of a well-known website accordingly. Providing PILs can also be useful for safety-netting. But do not just give a PIL as standard when it doesn't form part of a natural consultation.

Offer a PIL:

'I can also give you a leaflet on . . ., which explains some of the things we have discussed today, as well as other useful information. Would you like me to give you one of these?'

Or

Direct to a website:

'Do you have access to the Internet?'

If yes:

'What you might also find useful is the British Society of X website, which has a good range of leaflets on various aspects of . . ., or a more general website, like www.patient.co.uk.'

If a patient has a condition that may benefit from specialist nurse input you can say:

'Would you be able to come in and see our X (asthma, diabetes, cancer, etc.) specialist nurse who can spend a bit more time going through what kinds of . . . and go through your medication with you? Would you be able to do that?'

6.17. Take responsibility for any gaps in understanding shown by the patient

Take responsibility for any gaps in understanding shown by the patient, in order to spare their anxiety over appearing slow or stupid. The wording of this is very important.

Use phrases like:

'Is there anything I have said that I have not been clear about?'

'Is there anything about what I've just said that I wasn't clear about?'

'Is there anything I haven't explained clearly?'

These phrases are better than saying *'Is there anything you didn't understand?'* Although having essentially the same meaning, the first examples do not demean the patient in any way, whereas the latter example might be taken as an insult to their intelligence.

Respond appropriately when the patient asks you anything.

6.18. Deal with any extra issues

Ask about any extra complaints/problems/issues only when you have adequately finished dealing with the patient's PC.

'Is there anything else at all that you would like to ask me?'

However, you can invite questions at all times during the consultation.

If the patient has a second complaint and it is something you feel you cannot deal with adequately in the remaining time, then it is appropriate to say:

'Now, because this is important for you, it makes it important for me, and so that's something we certainly need to look at. I don't think we will have time today, but once this has settled, would it be okay to come back and see me and maybe we can look at it then?'

6.19. Close consultation

Close the consultation with a definitive end (closing farewell):

'Okay, Mr X. Thank you very much for coming. Here's your prescription.'

'Okay, Mr X. Thank you very much for coming. Here's your information leaflet, which you can take away with you to read.'

'Okay, Mr X. Thank you very much for coming. Here's your appointment for next time.'

Stand up.

Hand the patient the prescription script/PIL/appointment card/investigation request/medical certificate, etc.

Shake their hand.

Show them to the door.

END.

Summarising, safety-netting, arranging follow-up, offering further information, taking responsibility for any gaps in understanding shown by the patient and closing the consultation should take about 1 minute to complete.

After closing the consultation, don't forget to housekeep to take care of yourself.

Chapter 7

Difficult/Challenging consultations

Dealing with difficult patients, conflict between patients and doctors, ethical dilemmas and medico-legal issues can be extremely challenging for the doctor. Difficult/Challenging consultations, also known as primary care challenges, refer to clinical situations that are more sensitive and complex, including:

7.1. Managing a patient demanding antibiotics for a self-limiting viral illness

7.2. Managing a patient demanding an X-ray clinically not indicated

7.3. Breaking bad news: a structured approach

7.4. Ethical dilemma: conflicts of interest regarding driving and epilepsy

7.5. Risk assessment

   7.5.1. Assessment of risk to self

   7.5.2. Assessment of risk to others: assessing risk to a child in postnatal depression

   7.5.3. Assessment of risk to a patient after an overdose

7.6. Assessment of a psychotic patient

7.7. Counselling for smoking cessation

7.8. 'I want a PSA test': appropriate counselling

7.9. Explaining a procedure/investigation: a basic structure

These cases focus on the more difficult aspects of communication, and have been designed to help you handle complex consultations with patients sensitively. The cases give you the opportunity to undertake challenging interviews, and provide further practical preparation for managing such cases.

7.1. Managing a patient demanding antibiotics for a self-limiting viral illness

Explore the patient's ICE – ideas (find out why the patient wants antibiotics)

'Why do you want the antibiotics?'

Explore the patient's ICE – concerns (find out what the patient is worried about if they don't have antibiotics)

'If you don't have the antibiotics, what do you think will happen?'

Explore the patient's ICE – expectations (find out what the patient expects from the antibiotics)

'What do you think the antibiotics will do?'

Explain why the patient does not need antibiotics

'I appreciate that you have a lot of discomfort in your throat. I can see it is distressing for you. And because it's viral, it does not mean less discomfort for you than if it was bacterial.

I can see that you are upset and would like some antibiotics. The reason I feel that you should not have any antibiotics is that from everything you have said and everything that I've seen suggests that it is very likely that your illness is caused by a virus, and antibiotics don't work on viruses/colds.

So if I were to prescribe you antibiotics, I would be giving you medication that will give you no benefit but may harm you, because medicines carry with them some risks of side effects and harm like . . . nausea and diarrhoea.

I hope you will understand why it would be wrong of me to give you something that can't help you but may harm you.'

Remain firm, stand by your decisions and have confidence in your own clinical judgement backed up with rational reasons why.

7.2. Managing a patient demanding an X-ray clinically not indicated

Explore the patient's ICE – ideas (find out why the patient wants an X-ray)

'Why do you want this X-ray really badly?'

Explore the patient's ICE – concerns (find out what the patient is worried about if they don't have an X-ray)

'If you don't have the X-ray, what do you think will happen?'

Explore the patient's ICE – expectations (find out what the patient expects from an X-ray)

'What do you think the X-ray will show?'

Explain why the patient does not need an X-ray

'Now, you said earlier that you wanted an X-ray. The reason I'm not going to send you for an X-ray is that X-rays look at bones and joints and not muscles, and from what you have described and also from examining you, this is a problem in your muscles, and therefore an X-ray just won't show anything.

So if I were to send you for an X-ray, I would be sending you for something that will give you no benefit but may potentially harm you, because an X-ray of your back exposes your body to a large amount of radiation.

I hope you will understand why it would be wrong of me to send you for something that can't help you but may harm you.'

Again, remain firm, stand by your decisions and have confidence in your own clinical judgement backed up with rational reasons why.

7.3. Breaking bad news: a structured approach

In every medical specialty, bad, sad and difficult information must be given to patients and their families. An insensitive approach increases the distress of recipients of bad news, may exert a lasting impact on their ability to adapt and adjust, and can lead to anger and increased risk of litigation.

There are lots of good practice guidelines for breaking bad news to patients who you have found to have cancer or any life-limiting disease. The SPIKES protocol is a systematic, straightforward and practical framework consisting of six steps for delivering bad news to patients in any situation. It was described by Robert Buckman, a professor of oncology in Toronto.[5] It is used worldwide, principally in oncology and palliative care medicine but also by other specialities that often disclose unfavourable medical information to patients.

The six-step SPIKES protocol for delivering bad news:

- **S**etting up the interview
- **P**erception
- **I**nvitation
- **K**nowledge transfer
- **E**motions and **E**mpathy
- **S**trategy and **S**ummary

Setting up the interview: preparation

Talking to patients and their families can be one of the most difficult parts of your life as a doctor, but you can make it one of the most rewarding. Although this may set off panic alarms inside your head, there are a few key things that can really help.

Think about the setting/scene

Have you got some privacy? It is essential that discussions take place in a suitable environment, ideally a quiet, warm side room or consulting area where you won't be disturbed. Turn off your phone and/or hand over your bleep to a colleague so you aren't disturbed. There should be adequate seating for everyone. Also, have a box of tissues ready in case the patient becomes upset and you need to offer them a tissue.

Be prepared

Make sure you have got all the information about the events surrounding the bad news. You need to be fully aware of all aspects of the situation before beginning a discussion with a patient. It may be useful to go over the case notes carefully to remind yourself of exactly what has happened, what is happening now and what is going to happen.

Sit down

Never break bad news standing up. Standing when you are talking to someone can give the impression that you don't have much time and need to rush off somewhere else. Sitting down relaxes the patient. Also, try to be seated on the same level as your patient.

Availability of support

Have you got any support, such as a nurse? Try to bring a member of the nursing staff with you: someone who can stay afterwards and explain or reinforce anything that you said.

Honesty

Be honest – this is a must. Honesty is one of the factors that patients and relatives value the most when dealing with doctors. They need the truth to make their personal adjustments and their future plans. Make sure that you do not stray from the facts, and if you are unsure about something, never make it up. Instead, offer to find out the things you don't know or arrange another meeting.

Finally:

- At all times, be polite and patient
- Look attentive and calm, and don't look nervous
- Show you're caring
- Don't rush the patient
- Adopt an active listening mode, paying attention to every clue the patient gives you
- Explain the facts clearly

Once you are prepared, welcome the patient politely into the consultation room and introduce yourself:

'Hello, good morning, Mr/Mrs/Miss X. Nice to meet you. Please do take a seat.' (Show to the chair)

'My name's Dr X. I'm a GP registrar.'

'I hope you have not had to wait too long in the waiting area.' or *'I hope we have not kept you waiting too long, Mr X.'*

Open the consultation to address the patient's agenda: what they have come in for (which might be completely different from your agenda).

'What can I do for you today?'

Don't deal with what they have come in for (unless it is a clinical emergency), as this does not give them a warning shot that you have some bad news.

'Mr X, I appreciate you have come for your . . . but I'm not going to be able to do that today because I have got something far more important to discuss with you.'

Casually set the scene. Is there anyone who should be there that isn't? There are two reasons why you should involve significant others (but remember this should be the patient's choice). Firstly, the patient will be under great strain, and it is really helpful to have someone with you that you care about and that cares about you when you are receiving news that might be distressing. Secondly, it is a warning to the patient, especially when they know they have come for some test results, as you don't normally ask a patient if they would like someone to be with them during a consultation.

'Is there anyone you came in with today?'

'Would you like to have someone in with you?' or *'Is there anyone you would like to be here with you today?'*

If patient the asks, *'Why are you asking, doctor?'*, reply appropriately by saying, *'I've got some important news to talk to you about.'*

NOT

'I've got some bad/serious news to talk to you about.'

You could also ask them how they will get home, as this may be relevant after receiving some bad news:

> *'How are you getting home today?'*
> *'Are you driving?'*

Perception: assessing the patient's perceptions, ideas and concerns

Assess the patient's emotional state:

> *'How are you feeling today?'*

Use open questions to clarify the patient's understanding about what's going on: find out what they already know and what they think before you start to tell them what you know and what you think. The principle is 'ask before you tell'!

> *'I would just like to ask what you have been told already.'*
> *'What have you been told already?'*
> *'What have you been told about all this so far?'*

Explore the patient's ICE – ideas (about symptoms/results)

> *'What do you think this might be?'*
> > *'What do you think might be going on?'*
> > *'What do you think might be causing it?'*
> > *'What do you think might be causing your symptoms?'*
> > *'What did you think was going on with you when you felt this lump?'*
> > *'Do you know why we sent you for that test?'*
> > *'You say that you know that you have a spot on your X-ray. Do you have any ideas what might be causing it?'*

This strategy will help you establish a picture of how the patient perceives the situation so far.

Explore the patient's ICE – concerns (about symptoms/results)

> *'Is there anything about what's going on that's particularly worrying you?'*
> > *'Is there anything about these symptoms that's particularly worrying you?'*
> > *'You said/mentioned earlier on that you're worried about the pain. Is there anything about the pain that's particularly worrying you?'*

'*What would be your worst fear with these symptoms?*'

'*Are you worried that this might be something serious?*'

Allow the patient to air their concerns fully.

Based on this information you can tailor the bad news to the patient-held ideas and concerns.

Invitation: how much does the patient want to know?

Some patients prefer to know every little detail about their diagnosis, prognosis and details of their illness (including printouts), whereas others just like to know the basics at that moment (for example, just the diagnosis and what's going to happen next). It is important to find out how much information the patient wants to know. How much detail does the patient want you to go into?

'*I have got the results with me here today. I would just like to ask, how much detail you would like me to go into?*'

'*What I mean is that some people prefer to know all the details about what's going on, whereas others just like to know the basics. How do you feel?*'

'*Are you the kind of person who prefers to know all the details about what is going on?*'

'*How much information would you like me to give you about your diagnosis and treatment?*'

'*If it turns out to be something serious, how much detail would you like me to go into?*'

'*Some people like to know everything all in one go, whereas others prefer to go little by little. How do you feel?*'

'*Some people like to be fully involved in the decisions, whereas others just like to know what they need to know. How do you feel?*'

Knowledge transfer: sharing information with the patient

Once you know how much detail the patient would like, you should break the bad news to them gently in small chunks, explaining one thing at a time. Provide little bits of information slowly and give the patient time to process and absorb the news. Start with a small warning shot first to lessen the shock that can follow the disclosure of bad news and use intermediate words to build up to the bad news.

Mirror the patient's language, trying to use the same words they use. Using the same vocabulary as the patient aids understanding and helps make the patient aware that you have listened to what they have been saying. For example, if they say 'back passage', then you should also use the phrase 'back passage'.

Avoid medical jargon and technical terms/euphemisms that some patients do not understand, such as 'sample', 'tissue', 'biopsy', 'histology', 'metastasised', 'stage'. Instead, explain the facts clearly in appropriate language that the patient can understand. For example, an alternative to the jargon 'tissue'/'sample'/'biopsy' is 'piece' and an alternative to 'metastasised' is 'spread'.

The amount of information given should be directed by the patient.

'Would you like me to go over some details with you?' or *'I'll just go over some of the details with you, if that's okay?'*

'Let's take this one step at a time, shall we?'

Start with a small warning shot:

'I'm going to tell you something quite difficult now.'

'Unfortunately, the results of the scan were not what we hoped.' or *'Unfortunately, looking at the results of the scan, it is not what we hoped.'*

'I'm afraid/Unfortunately I've got some very bad news for you, Mr X.' or *'I'm afraid/Unfortunately I've got some very bad news to tell you, Mr X.'*

Use intermediate words to build up to the bad news:

'Mr X, I'm sorry to (have to) tell you that . . . we found something quite serious. We found a growth. It's what we call a tumour, and that tumour is a type of cancer.'

'I'm sorry to (have to) tell you that.'

Or

'The pieces they took from your X were looked at under the microscope, and I'm sorry to (have to) tell you that they did show something quite serious. There is a growth. It's what we call a tumour, and that tumour is a type of cancer.'

'I'm sorry to (have to) tell you that'

Then silence to allow time for the patient's emotion.

'I'm sorry to tell you that you have some form of cancer.'

Emotions and Empathy: responding to the patient's feelings

How a person responds to receiving bad news will be very personal. A patient's emotional reaction may vary from silence to disbelief, crying, shock, denial or anger. Everyone is different, and each person grieves in his or her own way. It is better to allow the patient to express their feelings of distress and pain. It is also important to recognise the patient's emotion, allow time for that emotion and respond appropriately, using reflection to demonstrate empathy and a caring manner.

Several examples of reflective/empathic statements/responses you can offer include:

'I can see this is very difficult/distressing for you.'

'I can see that you are upset.'

'I can see that you are upset hearing this news.'

'I can see that this has come as an awful shock/surprise to you.'

'I can see that this has caused you a lot of upset.'

'I can see that hearing the result/news of the scan is clearly a major shock to you.'

'You seem to be very upset by that.'

'You look really upset.'

'Hearing the result/news of the bone scan is clearly a major shock to you.'

'It must be difficult for you.'

Reassure the patient:

'Don't worry, cry as much as you need to, I am here to help you.'

'No, I don't think you are being silly. Anyone else would react like this in this situation.'

'It's a natural response to be upset. Anyone else would react like this in this situation.'

'I can see that you are upset hearing this news and it's a natural response to be upset. Anyone else would react like this in this situation.'

'I think that's an absolutely/perfectly normal response in someone in your situation. Other people in your situation would feel the same way.'

'I can see that this has made you feel angry, and it's okay for you to be angry at this time.'

If a patient shuts down or is completely shocked upon hearing the bad news – for example, if they put their hands around their head or they stop listening to anything you are saying – then stop talking and let there be silence, as this shows sensitivity to the patient's feelings. Don't say anything until they look up and are ready to continue.

If they don't talk for a while, ask:

'Mr X, what's going through your mind?' or *'Mr X, what are you thinking?'*

'Are you ready to carry on?'

'Is there somebody you would like me to call for you?'

'Is there any way I can make this better for you?'

Explore the patient's ICE – concerns (about the diagnosis)

'Is there anything about what's going on that's particularly worrying you?'

'Is there anything about hearing this diagnosis that's particularly worrying you?'

Strategy and Summary: planning the next step

Give the patient a clear strategy and plan for further care (what's going to happen next).

'I would like to move on to talk about what will happen next, if that's okay?'

Explain to the patient who else will be getting involved in the next step:

'What's going to happen next is that we will arrange an appointment for you to see the specialist at hospital next week. The cancer doctors will also go through more details with you.'

Follow-up

Arrange follow-up appointments in hospital and also with yourself. Schedule the next meeting as to when you want to see them again. Leave a means of contact if they want to follow up your discussion.

'I would like to see you the day after that, because you might have some questions.'

'This has obviously come as a big shock to you. Shall we arrange to meet again to go through things further? Shall we meet on . . . Friday at 2 p.m.? Is that a suitable time?'

'I appreciate that this is a lot of new information to take in. Between now and the hospital appointment, if you think of any questions, anything you're not sure about or need some advice, then write them down and bring them with you when you come to see me and we can go over them when we meet again.'

Leave emergency contact details (e.g. specialist nurse, secretary):

'Here are some emergency contact details of the . . . specialist nurse in case you need to ring us urgently.'

If appropriate, leave them with something hopeful:

'We will be doing our utmost to make this as easy for you as possible, Mr X.'

Summarise

Summarise the discussion, going over the key points you have been through so far: *'I know it's a lot to take in, but just to summarise, unfortunately we did find this cancer, but I want you to remember that . . .'*

Give the patient some time to collect their thoughts.

Further information: offer a PIL

'I can also give you a leaflet on . . ., which explains some of the things we have discussed today, as well as other useful information. Would you like me to give you one of these?'

Take responsibility for any gaps in understanding shown by the patient

'Is there anything I have said that I have not been clear about?'

Leave time for the patient to ask questions:

'Is there anything else at all that you would like to ask me?'

Close consultation

'Okay, Mr X.'

'I'll just give you your information leaflet, which you can take away with you to read.'

Stand up.

Hand the patient the PIL/appointment card/emergency contact details, etc.

Shake their hand.

Show them to the door.

7.4. Ethical dilemma: conflicts of interest regarding driving and epilepsy

A 28-year-old female with epilepsy, which has been well-controlled with anticonvulsant therapy for 10 years, has had a recent fit. She has come to see you 2 weeks later, and your task is to tell her that one of the things she is unable to do is to drive anymore for 1 year.

Introduce yourself to the patient, using your professional title and surname:

'Hello, good morning, Mrs X. Nice to meet you. Please do take a seat.'

(Show to the chair)

'My name's Dr X, I'm a GP registrar.'

Try to establish rapport:

'We have not met before, have we? Well, it's lovely to meet you.'

Open the consultation:

'What can I do for you today?' or *'I understand you recently had a fit after many years.'*

'Oh, I'm sorry to hear that.'

'Can you tell me more about that, please?'

Counsel the patient about driving and epilepsy:

'Has anyone informed you of anything that you must not do because you have had a fit?'

If yes:

'How do you feel about that?'

If no:

'Do you drive?'

'I'm going to tell you something quite difficult now.'

'Unfortunately, because you have had an epileptic fit, I hope you will understand that you must not do anything that if you have a fit will put yourself or other people at danger.'

'What this means is that one of the things you won't be able to do is to drive anymore for 1 year.'

'I'm sorry to have to tell you that.'

'How do you feel about that?'

'The law is very clear on this.'

'I can see this is very difficult for you.' or 'I can see this has come as an awful shock to you.'

'I think that's an absolutely normal response in someone in your situation. Other people in your situation would feel the same way.'

'You did the right thing coming today.'

'I hope you will understand that if you do drive, not only will you be putting yourself at risk but also other people are at risk of being harmed.'

'It is also extremely important to let the DVLA know about your recent fit, and it is your responsibility to contact and inform the DVLA.'

'If you continue to drive, as I've tried to explain, not only are you putting yourself at risk but also other people, and I am obliged/it's my obligation to pass this information on to the DVLA.'

'I'm sorry to have to tell you that.'

'If you fail to inform the DVLA, then I'm afraid I'm going to have to contact the DVLA myself (today), and what that means is your licence may be revoked and also you could get in trouble with the law, as you have a duty to inform them.'

'I'm sorry to have to tell you that.'

'I hope you will understand why I have a professional responsibility to contact the DVLA myself if you don't do this.'

'Is there anything about hearing this news that's particularly worrying you?'

'Once you are free from a fit for . . . a year, we can review the whole situation and you should be able to drive again.'

'I can see this is very difficult for you.'

Patient education:

'I would like to ask you a couple more things, if that's okay?'

'How did you get here today?'

'Unfortunately, you won't be able to drive home.'

'Would you be able to ask someone to come and pick you up?'

'Other things you won't be able to do for the time being are things like swimming on your own, cycling at busy times, and climbing ladders, trees or scaffolding, such that if you were to have a fit you would be likely to hurt yourself or others.'

'Is there anything you would like me to go over again?'

Check compliance:

'It would help me if I knew more about your medication.'

'Are you taking your medication?'

'How do you take your medication?'

'It's very important that you take these tablets at the right time every day.'

'It is extremely important that you don't drink alcohol with them.'

'If you go anywhere, you must take them with you.'

'I would like to ask you a couple more things, if that's okay?'

'Are you currently sexually active?'

'At some point, we will need to discuss regular contraception with you. These tablets can interfere with the Pill and make it less active. Therefore, other precautions would be needed, such as condoms, which also have the advantage of protecting against sexually transmitted diseases.'

'Pregnancy will need to be planned. Some of the drugs we use can harm the baby. If you want to have a baby, you must come back and see me to review the whole situation.'

'Finally, about career planning, there are certain things you won't be able to do, such as be a pilot or a heavy goods vehicle driver.'

Further information: offer a PIL:

'I can also give you a leaflet on epilepsy and driving, which explains some of the things we have discussed today, as well as other useful information. Would you like me to give you one of these?'

Take responsibility for any gaps in understanding shown by the patient:

'Is there anything I have said that I have not been clear about?'

Leave time for the patient to ask questions:

'Is there anything else at all that you would like to ask me?'

Close consultation:

'Okay, Mrs X.'

'I'll just give you your information leaflet, which you can take away with you to read.'

'If you have any questions, do come back and see me again.'

Stand up.

Hand the patient the PIL.

Shake their hand.

Show them to the door.

7.5. Risk assessment

Retrospective studies have shown that in half of all suicides, the individual had seen their GP in the preceding 4 weeks.[6] So, a key issue is identifying those who are or might be considering suicide.

It is important to approach issues regarding risk of deliberate self-harm, risk of suicide and risk of harm to others sensitively. Although there are a number of tools that can be used in assessing risk, mostly in the form of questionnaires, it remains very difficult. There are, however, some general principles that can help in allowing patients to express their intentions.

The next three cases go through how to conduct an assessment of risk in primary care to help you to identify patients who are at risk of harm to self or others so that you can plan their care: that may be in the community with support from a psychiatrist, community psychiatric nurse or other organisation or inpatient care – voluntarily or on section. The first case looks at the systematic assessment of risk to self, the second looks at the assessment of risk to others (using risk to a child in postnatal depression as an example) and the third looks at how to assess risk in a patient who has taken an overdose.

7.5.1. Assessment of risk to self

This section looks at how to systematically assess risk of DSH and suicide in primary care.

The systematic assessment of suicidal risk:

◆ Ask how the patient is feeling at the moment

◆ Ask about the patient's mood

◆ Ask when they felt at their worst, if they ever had any thoughts about harming themselves or ending their life (suicide)

◆ If yes, ask whether they have made any plans to act on their thoughts/ feelings of ending their life

◆ If yes, ask whether they have made any final preparations

Introduce yourself to the patient, using your professional title and surname:

'Hello, good morning, Mr/Mrs/Miss X. Nice to meet you. Please do take a seat.' (Show to the chair)

'My name's Dr X. I'm a GP registrar.'

Try to establish rapport:

'We have not met before, have we? Well, it's lovely to meet you.'

Warn/Signpost to the patient that you will be asking some personal/sensitive questions:

'I would like to ask you a few personal questions, if that's okay?' or *'As it's relevant and may be important, I'd like to ask some sensitive questions, if that's okay?'*

Then systematically and sensitively undertake the assessment of risk to self:

Ask how the patient is feeling at the moment

Start the risk assessment gently by asking how they are feeling, and build up very quickly.

'How are you feeling at the moment?' or *'How do you feel within yourself?'*

'Oh, I'm sorry to hear that.'

'Can you tell me a little bit more about that, please?'

Ask about the patient's mood

'I would like to know if there have been any times when you have felt particularly low.'

Ask when they felt at their worst, if they ever had any thoughts about harming themselves or ending their life (suicide)

Introduce the topic using normalising statements, and then move on to find out whether there is a wish to self-harm or end their life. This needs to be done tactfully but directly.

'Sometimes, when people are feeling low, they have thoughts that perhaps life is not worth living anymore, if it were to continue as it is at the moment, or they have thoughts about harming themselves. Have you ever had these thoughts/have you ever felt like that?'

Or

'Have there been any times when you have felt that life might not be worth living, if it were to continue as it is at the moment?'

Note: It is a fallacy that raising the issue of suicide will either provoke someone who is considering it, or someone who hasn't previously thought about it, to act.

If yes, ask whether they have made any plans to act on their thoughts/feelings of ending their life

If there is a wish to self-harm or end their life, find out whether they have made any plans to act on their thoughts/feelings.

'Obviously that's quite a distressing thought to have.'

'I can see this is very difficult for you.' (Reflection)

'It's actually not that uncommon for people to feel like this when they are depressed. So you're not alone in terms of the feelings you have had.'

'How often are you having these thoughts?'

'Now, when you have had that kind of thought come to mind, have you actually thought of ways in which you may go about harming yourself?' or *'When that thought has come to mind, have you thought of what you might actually do?'* or *'Have you made any plans of how you might go about harming yourself?'*

'Can you tell me a little bit more about that, please?'

'Can I ask how strong the feeling is to harm yourself?'

If yes, ask whether they have made any final preparations

'Sometimes, people feeling this desperate may write a note or make sure that their will is up-to-date. Have you made any final preparations or acts?'

Use closed questions to clinch details of the risk assessment

'Have you ever thought of other ways of harming yourself apart from . . . taking a drug overdose?'

> *'Have you ever done anything to hurt yourself in the past?'*
>
> *'Have you ever taken an overdose in the past?'*
>
> *'What is the most tablets you have ever taken?'*
>
> *'How do you feel about the future?'* or *'How do you see the future?'*

7.5.2. Assessment of risk to others: assessing risk to a child in postnatal depression

This section looks at how to systematically assess risk of harm to others in primary care.

An approach to the assessment of risk to others in primary care, using risk to a child in postnatal depression as an example:

Warn/Signpost to the patient that you will be asking some personal/sensitive questions:

'Again, I need to ask you some questions in relation to your child.'

Deal sensitively with issues regarding risk of harm to others. Introduce the topic using normalising statements.

'Sometimes, when people are feeling particularly low, how they feel about their child is also affected. How have you been feeling about your child?'

If the patient asks:

'What do you mean, doctor?'

Respond appropriately by saying:

'Sometimes, when people are feeling low, they don't have the normal sense of affection and warmth towards their child. Have you felt like that?'

If yes:

'Do you blame yourself and feel guilty about it?'

'Given the way you feel for the baby, have you felt as if you may harm the baby?'

If yes:

'Obviously, that's quite a distressing thought to have.'

'How often do these thoughts come to mind?'

'Now, when you have had that kind of thought come to mind, have you actually thought of ways in which you may go about harming your baby?' or *'When that thought has come to mind, have you thought of what you might actually do?'* or

'Have you made any plans of how you might go about harming your baby?'

'Can you tell me a little bit more about that, please?'

'Can I ask how strong the feeling is to harm your baby?'

7.5.3. Assessment of risk to a patient after an overdose

This section looks at how to assess risk in a patient who has taken an overdose in primary care.

The systematic assessment of risk in a patient who has taken an overdose:

Introduce yourself to the patient, using your professional title and surname:

'Hello, good morning, Mr/Mrs/Miss X. Nice to meet you. Please do take a seat.'
(Show to the chair)

'My name's Dr X. I'm a GP registrar.'

Try to establish rapport:

'We have not met before, have we? Well, it's lovely to meet you.'

Undertake the assessment of risk to self:

'I understand you were recently in hospital because you took some tablets. Can you tell me a little bit more about that, please?'

'Was it something that you had been thinking about for quite some time?'

'Can I ask how strong the feeling was to harm yourself?'

'Sometimes, people feeling this desperate may write a note or make sure their will is up-to-date. Did you make any final preparations or acts?'

'How are you feeling at the moment?'

'Do you feel frightened?'

Use closed questions to clinch details of the risk assessment:

'Have you ever thought of other ways of harming yourself apart from . . . taking a drug overdose?'

'Have you ever done anything else to hurt yourself in the past?'

'Have you ever taken an overdose in the past?'

'What is the most tablets you have ever taken?'

'How do you feel about the future?' or 'How do you see the future?'

'Is it something you may try again?'

'Have you ever suffered from depression?'

'Have you ever been on any tablets for depression?'

Then assess the core characteristic:

- Low mood
- Anhedonia (loss/lack of interest, enjoyment or pleasure)
- Anergia (loss/lack of energy)

Low mood

'During the last month, have you been feeling particularly down/low, depressed or hopeless?'

'I would like to know if there have been any times during the last month when you have been feeling particularly down/low, depressed or hopeless?'

'I would like to know if there have been any times when you have felt particularly down/low, depressed or hopeless?'

Anhedonia (loss of interest, enjoyment or pleasure)

'During the last month, have you lost interest, enjoyment or pleasure in doing things?'

'During the last month, have you often been bothered by having little interest, enjoyment or pleasure in doing things?'

'Do you still enjoy the things you used to enjoy doing?'

'Is there anything that you are able to get enjoyment out of?'

Anergia (lack of energy)

'During the last month, have you often been bothered by feeling tired or had little energy?'

If a patient answers yes to any of these questions (low mood, anhedonia or anergia), enquire about any secondary/accessory (biological and cognitive) symptoms of depression, such as reduced concentration and attention, reduced self-esteem and self-confidence, feelings of worthlessness or guilt, disturbed sleep, loss of interest in sex (loss of libido), diminished appetite and weight loss, to establish the severity of the patient's depression.

Reduced concentration and attention

'During the last month, have you often been bothered by poor concentration?'

'During the last month, have you often been bothered by trouble concentrating on things, such as reading the newspaper or watching television?'

Reduced self-esteem and self-confidence

'During the last month, have you often been bothered by low self-esteem and self-confidence?'

Feelings of worthlessness or guilt

'During the last month, have you often been bothered by feelings of worthlessness or guilt?'

Disturbed sleep

'During the last month, have you often been bothered by trouble falling or staying asleep, or sleeping too much?'

Loss of interest in sex

'During the last month, have you often been bothered by loss of interest in sex?'

Diminished appetite

'During the last month, have you often been bothered by poor appetite or overeating?'

'Have there been any changes in your appetite?'

'How's your appetite?'

Weight loss

'Have there been any changes in your weight?'

7.6. Assessment of a psychotic patient

When assessing a psychotic patient, introduce the topic using normalising statements so that the patient doesn't feel it's just them, but that it's part of everyday routine practice.

'I would like to ask you a routine question that we ask everybody.'

Or

'Sometimes, people feeling like this . . .'

Enquire about the following psychotic symptoms:

Auditory hallucinations

'I would like to ask you a routine question that we ask everybody. Do you ever seem to hear noises or voices when there is no one about and nothing else to explain them?'

Or

'Sometimes, people feeling like this hear noises or voices when there is no one about and nothing else to explain them. Has this ever happened to you?'
'What is it like?'
'What do you hear?'
'Do the voices you hear ever talk about you?'
'Do the voices you hear ever give a running commentary on what you are doing?

Other hallucinations

'Do you have similar experiences with strange sights, smells or tastes?'

Persecutory delusions

'Do you ever think people are deliberately trying to harm or kill you?'

Delusions of reference

'Do you ever feel that messages are specifically intended for you?'

Origins of delusions

'How did these ideas come into your mind?'

    'What is the explanation for this?'

Intensity of delusion

'Even when you seem most convinced, do you really feel in the back of your mind that it might not be true?'

7.7. Counselling for smoking cessation

Guidance for encouraging smoking cessation in general practice[7,8]:

1. Ask
2. Advise
3. Assess
4. Assist
5. Arrange

'Now, while you are here, do you have a few minutes? I just wanted to discuss one or two other things with you.'

1. Ask

Ask about smoking status indirectly or directly.

Indirectly, for example, if the patient presents with worsening asthma:

'What do you think caused the asthma attack?'

'Do you think smoking is affecting your asthma?'

Directly:

'Do you smoke?' or *'You said earlier that you smoke?'*

Nicotine addiction can be assessed by:

- The number of cigarettes smoked per day
- The time taken before lighting the first cigarette (wake-to-light time)[9]

Smoking >15 cigarettes per day and wake-to-light time of <30 minutes suggests significant nicotine dependence.[7]

'How many do you smoke a day?'

'How long have you been smoking?' or *'When did you start to smoke?'*

'When you wake up in the morning, how long is it before you have the first cigarette?'

Other useful questions you can ask include:

'Under what circumstances do you smoke?'

'Does anybody else at home or work smoke?'

2. **Advise**

Advise on the benefits of stopping smoking in a personalised and appropriate way.

'Have you had any thoughts about smoking and your general health?'

'Do you know any risks associated with smoking?'

'Do you know of any benefits of stopping smoking?'

'People who smoke are more likely to have heart attacks, strokes, lung disease, etc.'

'The evidence shows that half of all smokers will die of smoking-related diseases.'

3. **Assess**

Assess the patient's motivation to stop smoking.

'Have you ever thought about stopping smoking?'

'Have you ever tried stopping in the past?'

If they have not tried stopping in the past:

'Would you like to stop smoking?'

If no:

'What is stopping you from giving up now?'

If yes:

'What is motivating you to stop now?'

'Are you aware of any treatments to help you stop smoking?'

'Are you aware of any treatments other than nicotine replacement therapy (NRT) to help you stop smoking?'

If they have tried stopping in the past, you need to review their past history of what helped and hindered:

'What did you do when you tried to stop?'

If they have tried NRT:

'Did you have any problems with NRT?'

'What made you start again?'

4. **Assist**

Assist the patient to stop smoking by offering support and NRT, bupropion (Zyban) or varenicline (Champix), where indicated.

'*There are a number of ways we can help you stop smoking. These include providing essential advice and support, NRT or some medication.*'

'*Can you tell me, is this something you have heard of before?*' or '*Have you heard about NRT before?*'

'*With regards to NRT, many products are available, such as patches, gums, inhalators/inhalers, lozenges, micro-tabs and nasal sprays.*'

'*NRT does not increase the risk of heart attacks and strokes.*'

'*We also have a smoking cessation clinic, which has an experienced counsellor who offers help and support, useful strategies to avoid temptation/relapse, as well as NRT and much more.*'

'*If you're interested, please take a leaflet or book/make an appointment at reception.*'

'*Finally, there are many independent, recommended support organisations/ services that provide essential support. The most well-known is Quitline. Again, if you're interested, please take a leaflet.*'

Quitline 0800 002 200, website www.quit.org.uk

---

5. **Arrange**

Arrange follow-up.

The patient must set a quit date.

'*I would like you to come back and see me in . . ., if that's okay?*'

Stand up.

Hand the patient the prescription/PIL/appointment card.

Shake their hand.

Show them to the door.

7.8. 'I want a PSA test': appropriate counselling

Introduce yourself to the patient, using your professional title and surname:

'Hello, good morning, Mr X. Nice to meet you. Please do take a seat.'

(Show to the chair)

'My name's Dr X, I'm a GP registrar.'

Try to establish rapport:

'We have not met before, have we? Well, it's lovely to meet you.'

Open the consultation:

'What can I do for you today?' or *'I understand you would like to have a PSA test.'*

'It would help me if I knew some of the reasons why you want the PSA test.'

Explore the patient's ICE – ideas about a PSA test (find out what the patient knows about a PSA test and why they want the test)

'What do you know about a PSA test?'

'Do you know what a high PSA means?'

'Do you know what a low PSA means?'

'Why do you want a PSA test?'

Explore the patient's ICE – concerns about a PSA test (find out what the patient is worried about having a PSA test)

'Is there anything about having this test that's particularly worrying you?'

'What would be your worst fear with a PSA test?'

Undertake a focused history and clinical examination of the patient

'Is it okay if I ask you a few questions that might be related to your prostate?'

◆ Enquire about the presence of any urinary symptoms: obstructive symptoms (hesitancy, poor stream, terminal dribbling and poor emptying) and irritable bladder symptoms (frequency, nocturia, urgency and urge incontinence) and the effect on the patient's quality of life due to symptoms

◆ Identify any red flags (appetite, weight loss, haematuria, bone pain, etc.)

◆ Explore the patient's ICE, PMH, DH, FH, PSH, etc.

◆ Perform a selective physical examination of the patient (abdominal and prostate)

Counsel the patient appropriately for a PSA test

Your discussion should include information about the prostate gland, prostate cancer and the PSA test itself.

'*Would you like me to go over some details about the PSA test with you?*' or '*I'll just go over some of the details about the PSA test with you, if that's okay?*'

'*Let's take this one step at a time, shall we?*'

'*Firstly, we will talk a bit about the prostate gland, then about prostate cancer and, finally, details about the PSA test itself.*'

The prostate gland:

'*The prostate gland is only found in men. It lies just under the bladder. The tube that passes urine from the bladder to the outside runs through the middle of the prostate.*'

Note: You can draw an image of this if you feel it will help explain this better to the patient.

'*The main function of the prostate gland is to produce fluid that helps produce healthy sperm.*'

'*The prostate gets bigger/enlarges gradually after the age of about 50. As the prostate enlarges, it may cause narrowing of the first part of the tube that passes urine from the bladder.*'

'*This can lead to some of the symptoms you have been experiencing.*'

'*Is there anything that you would like to ask me about this?*'

Prostate cancer:

'*We will now move on to talk about prostate cancer.*'

'*Prostate cancer is common and is the second most common cause of cancer deaths in men in the UK.*'

'The average age of diagnosis is between 70 and 74 years. It is less common in men under the age of 50 years.'

'Some people are more likely to get it than others. It is more common in people who have a FH (of prostate cancer)/family member with prostate cancer or who are Afro-Caribbean.'

'Prostate cancer can grow slowly or very quickly. Slow-growing cancers are common and may not cause any symptoms or shorten life.'

'There is no evidence that detection of early prostate cancer leads to longer survival.'

'Is there anything that you would like to ask me?'

The PSA test:

'Okay, we will now move on to talk about the PSA test.'

'The PSA test is a blood test that measures the level of PSA in your blood.'

'PSA is made by the prostate gland, and some of it will leak into your blood depending on your age and the health of your prostate.'

'A raised PSA level may mean you have prostate cancer. However, other conditions, such as age-related enlargement of the prostate (sometimes called benign prostatic hyperplasia), infection of the prostate (prostatitis) and urinary infection, can also cause a high PSA.'

'It is important to realise that about two out of three men with a raised PSA level will not have prostate cancer. And a normal PSA does not mean you do not have prostate cancer. One in five men with a normal PSA will have cancer. So, the PSA test can miss cancer.'

'Also, the test cannot distinguish between aggressive and slow-growing cancers and may detect cancer that would not otherwise become evident in your life.'

'When you have a PSA test, you should not have had a water infection in the last month, ejaculated or exercised heavily in the last 48 hours, had a prostate biopsy in the last 6 weeks or had a rectal examination in the last week, as each of these may produce an unusually high PSA result.'

'After you have had a PSA test, . . .

. . . *if your PSA level is not raised*, you are unlikely to have cancer and no immediate further action is needed.'

. . . if your PSA level is slightly raised, you probably do not have cancer, but you might need further tests, including more PSA tests.'

. . . if your PSA level is definitely raised, we will arrange for you to see a specialist for further tests to find out if you have prostate cancer.'

'Because this test is not specific for prostate cancer, all patients with a very high PSA should have a prostate biopsy.'[10]

Summarise

Summarise the discussion, going over the key points you have been through so far.

'I know it's a lot to take in, but just to summarise, the important points that I want you to remember are . . .'

Further information: offer a PIL

'I can also give you a leaflet on the PSA test, which explains some of the things we have discussed today, as well as other useful information. Would you like me to give you one of these?'

Take responsibility for any gaps in understanding shown by the patient

'Is there anything I have said that I have not been clear about?'

'Is there anything else at all that you would like to ask me?'

Close consultation

'Okay, Mr X.'

'I'll just give you your information leaflet, which you can take away with you to read.'

Stand up.

Hand the patient the investigation request/PIL.

Shake their hand.

Show them to the door.

7.9. Explaining a procedure/investigation: a basic structure

Points to consider in your discussion when explaining a procedure/investigation to a patient – useful if you get stuck!

- Explore patient's health beliefs (ICE) – ideas about investigation
- Explore patient's health beliefs (ICE) – ideas about diagnosis
- Explore patient's health beliefs (ICE) – concerns about diagnosis
- Inform patient of investigation
- Explore patient's understanding of investigation
- Explain investigation:
  - Preparation
  - Description
  - Important side effects and risks
  - Results
- Explore patient's health beliefs (ICE) – concerns about investigation
- Further management
- Summarise
- Further information: offer a PIL
- Take responsibility for any gaps in understanding shown by the patient
- Close consultation

An example using an endoscopy is provided following to practically illustrate this simple structure for explaining a procedure to the patient.

Introduce yourself to the patient, using your professional title and surname:

'Hello, good morning, Mr/Mrs/Miss X. Nice to meet you. Please do take a seat.'

(Show to the chair)

'My name's Dr X, I'm a GP registrar.'

Try to establish rapport:

'We have not met before, have we? Well, it's lovely to meet you.'

Open the consultation:

'What can I do for you today?' or *'I understand you are having a . . . endoscopy.'*

Explore patient's health beliefs (ICE) – ideas about investigation

'Do you know why we are doing/you are having this test?'

'The reason we are doing this test is because you have been having problems with . . . your stomach.'

Explore patient's health beliefs (ICE) – ideas about diagnosis

'What do you think might be causing your symptoms?'

'In terms of the pain, have you had any thoughts as to what's going on?'

'Have you had any thoughts as to what's causing your symptoms?'

'Have you had any thoughts as to what this might be?'

'Have you talked to your friends or family? What do they think it is?'

Explore patient's health beliefs (ICE) – concerns about diagnosis

'Is there anything about these symptoms that's particularly worrying you?'

'Is there anything about what's going on that's particularly worrying you?'

'You said earlier on that you're worried about the pain. Is there anything about the pain that's particularly worrying you?'

'What would be your worst fear with these symptoms?'

'Are you worried that this might be something serious?'

Inform patient of investigation

'The test is called . . . an endoscopy.'

 'Can you tell me, is this test something you have heard of before?'

Explore patient's understanding of investigation

'What do you know about having a . . . endoscopy?'

 'Would you like me to go over some details with you?' or *'I'll just go over some of the details with you, if that's okay?'*

 'Let's take this one step at a time, shall we?'

Explain investigation – preparation

Firstly, explain what they will need to do practically to prepare for the procedure, for example, just turn up, have a full bladder, don't eat for X hours before the planned test.

 'An endoscopy is usually done as an outpatient/day case to look at your food pipe/gullet, stomach and first part of your gut.'

 'What you need to do to prepare for this test is . . . you should not eat or drink for 4–6 hours before the test. Small sips of water may be allowed up to 2 hours before the test.'

 'This is really important because if you do then they won't be able to perform the test and it will have to be cancelled.'

 'Some of your medication may need to be stopped before the test.'

Explain investigation – description

Go through the specific details of what will happen on the day, whether they will be awake/asleep, if it will be painful, how long the procedure will take, etc.

 'An endoscope is a thin flexible telescope. It is about as thick as your little finger. It contains a tiny camera to look inside your gut.'

 'What's going to happen when you go for this test . . . your endoscopy . . . is they may give you a numbing spray to the back of the throat, so that it's not as uncomfortable. They may also give you some medicine to relax you, but it can make you feel sleepy/drowsy and forgetful. But you won't actually be asleep because they will ask you to swallow the first part of the endoscope.'

 'When they are doing this test and looking at your food pipe, stomach and first

part of your gut, they might take a very small piece(s) from each of these three areas to look at in the lab to find out why this is happening.'

'I would recommend that you . . .'

Don't use words/euphemisms such as 'sedative'/'sedated', 'biopsy'/'tissue'/'samples' or 'cytology'/'histology'.

Explain investigation – important side effects and risks

Make the patient aware of the relative risks/complications of the procedure.

'Everyone usually has a sore throat for a few days, and they may give you some painkillers for this.'

'There is a very small risk of there being some damage to the blood vessels, and therefore some bleeding and a small risk of damage to the gullet/stomach during the procedure. Usually, they can deal with it at the time. The person doing the procedure will go through this with you in more detail before you have the test.'

Explain investigation – results

Inform the patient when to expect the results of the test. If the patient knows it takes 2 weeks beforehand, you're helping to manage expectations, and avoiding unnecessary anxiety and worry.

'Some of the results they will be able to tell you straight away on the same day. They may be able to tell you if you have a stomach bug. The majority/rest of the results usually take at least 2 weeks to come back, as they have to send them to a lab to look at under a microscope. When the results are back, please do come back and I will discuss/go through them with you then.'

Explore patient's health beliefs (ICE) – concerns about investigation

'Is there anything about having this test that's particularly worrying you?'

Further management

Explain what might happen when the results are back.

'Depending on what we find, you may need to have . . . further tests, some medicine(s) to . . . or see a specialist.'

'If there is anything else, then we will discuss that once we have the results because we don't know what's going on at the moment.'

'Why don't we discuss these when we have all of the results?'

Summarise

'I know it's a lot to take in, but just to summarise, the important points that I want you to remember are . . .'

Further information: offer a PIL

'I can also give you a leaflet on . . . an endoscopy, which explains some of the things we have discussed today, as well as other useful information. Would you like me to give you one of these?'

Or

Direct to a website:

'Do you have access to the Internet?'

If yes:

'What you might also find useful is the British Society of X website, which has a good range of leaflets on various aspects of . . ., or a more general website, like www.patient.co.uk.'

If a patient has a condition that may benefit from specialist nurse input, you can say:

'Would you be able to come in and see our X specialist nurse who can spend a bit more time going through what kinds of . . . and go through your medication with you? Would you be able to do that?'

Take responsibility for any gaps in understanding shown by the patient

'Is there anything I have said that I have not been clear about?'

'Is there anything else at all that you would like to ask me?'

Close consultation

'Okay, Mr X. Thank you very much for coming. Here's your information leaflet, which you can take away with you to read.'

Stand up.

    Hand the patient the PIL.

    Shake their hand.

    Show them to the door.

References

1. Riley B, Haynes J, Field S. *The Condensed Curriculum Guide for GP Training and the New MRCGP*. London: Royal College of General Practitioners; 2007.

2. Neighbour R. *The Inner Consultation: how to develop an effective and intuitive consulting style*. 2nd ed. Oxford: Radcliffe Publishing; 2004.

3. National Institute for Health and Clinical Excellence (NICE). Depression with a Chronic Physical Health Problem: NICE guideline 91. London: NICE; 2011. www.nice.org.uk/guidance/CG91

4. Zigmond AS, Snaith RP. The hospital anxiety and depression scale. *Acta Psychiatr Scand*. 1983; **67**(6): 361–70.

5. Baile WF, Buckman R, Lenzi R, *et al*. SPIKES – A six-step protocol for delivering bad news: application to the patient with cancer. *Oncologist*. 2000; **5**(4): 302–11.

6. Vassilas CA, Morgan HG. General practitioners' contact with victims of suicide. *BMJ*. 1993; **307**(6899): 300–1.

7. Fowler G. Helping smokers to stop: an evidence-based approach. *Practitioner*. 2000; **244**(1606): 37–41.

8. British Heart Foundation. *Stopping Smoking: evidence-based guidance*. Factfile 8/2001. London: British Heart Foundation; n.d.

9. Moxham J. Nicotine addiction. *BMJ*. 2000; **320**(7232): 391–2.

10. Burford D, Austoker J, Kirby M. *PSA Testing for Prostate Cancer*. Available at: www.patient.co.uk/health/PSA-Testing-for-Prostate-Cancer.htm (accessed 12 January 2012).

Index